2nd Edition

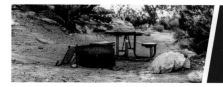

BEST ⚕ TENT
Camping

UTAH

YOUR CAR-CAMPING GUIDE TO SCENIC BEAUTY, THE SOUNDS
OF NATURE, AND AN ESCAPE FROM CIVILIZATION

For Jane, my faithful companion

Best of Tent Camping: Utah
Copyright © 2017 by Jeffrey Steadman
All rights reserved
Published by Menasha Ridge Press
Printed in the United States of America
Distributed by Publishers Group West
Second edition, first printing

Library of Congress Cataloging-in-Publication Data

Names: Steadman, Jeffrey, author.
Title: The best in tent camping. Utah : your car-camping guide to scenic beauty, the sounds of nature, and an escape
   from civilization / by Jeffrey Steadman.
Description: Second edition. | Birmingham, Alabama : Menasha Ridge Press, [2017] | "Distributed by Publishers Group
   West"
   —T.p. verso. | Includes index.
Identifiers: LCCN 2017014095 | ISBN 978-1-63404-072-3 (paperback : alk. paper) | ISBN 978-1-63404-073-0 (e-book)
Subjects: LCSH: Campsites, facilities, etc.—Utah—Directories. | Camping—Utah—Guidebooks. | Utah—Guidebooks.
Classification: LCC GV191.42.U8 S74 2017 | DDC 796.5409792—dc23
LC record available at lccn.loc.gov/2017014095

Project editor: Ritchey Halphen
Cover design: Scott McGrew
Maps: Steve Jones and Jeffrey Steadman
Book design: Jonathan Norberg
Photos: Jeffrey Steadman, except where noted
Copy editor: Susan Roberts McWilliams
Proofreader: Vanessa Lynn Rusch
Indexer: Rich Carlson

MENASHA RIDGE PRESS
An imprint of AdventureKEEN
2204 First Ave. S., Ste. 102
Birmingham, AL 35233

Visit menasharidge.com for a complete listing of our books and for ordering information. Contact us at our website, at
facebook.com/menasharidge, or at twitter.com/menasharidge with questions or comments. To find out more about
who we are and what we're doing, visit blog.menasharidge.com.

Front cover: The unique rock formations of Goblin Valley State Park (see page 132); photo: Jeffrey Steadman

2nd Edition

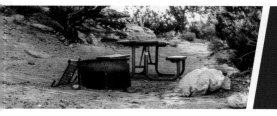

BEST TENT Camping

UTAH

YOUR CAR-CAMPING GUIDE TO SCENIC BEAUTY, THE SOUNDS
OF NATURE, AND AN ESCAPE FROM CIVILIZATION

Jeffrey Steadman

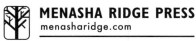

MENASHA RIDGE PRESS
menasharidge.com

Your Guide to the Outdoors Since 1982

Utah Campground Locator Map

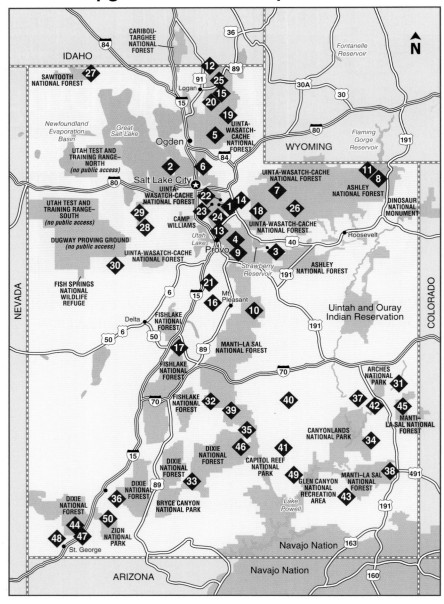

CONTENTS

Map Legend

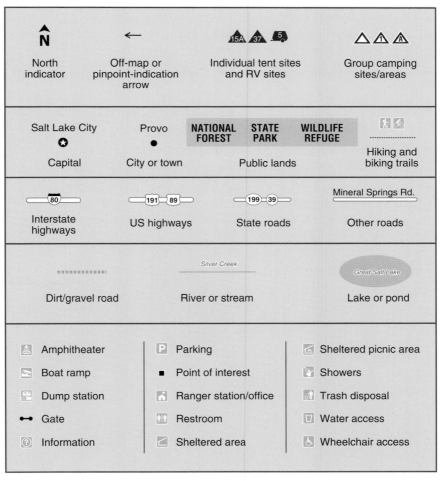

ACKNOWLEDGMENTS

I would like to thank the following humans (and one nonhuman):

- All of those puzzled campground hosts, forest rangers, land managers, and wary locals who answered my unending questions and strange requests this time around. Fortunately, kindness has not gone out of style since the first edition of this book was published.

- Everyone at AdventureKEEN for trusting me once again with the task of camping up and down this state and turning my notes and scribbles into this slick book you now hold in your hands.

- My father, Kerry, for instilling in me a love of the outdoors in the first place. Without him, there would be no book.

- My family—my mother, Robyn; siblings Jenn, Rick, Greg, and Scott; and Uncle Gary for checking in on me and cheering me on.

- Everyone in my Yelp family, for allowing me to bring the outdoors into my day job, and for giving me the means to keep on camping.

- And, finally, the Jane Dog, the greatest camping partner I could ever wish for and a true companion. She's trekked over some rough terrain with me and never left my side, not just on sunny days, but through the pouring rain. Now *that's* true loyalty.

To all of you—*thanks*.

—Jeffrey Steadman

PREFACE

People often ask me, "What's your favorite campground?"

That would be like asking a mother to pick her favorite child: it really depends on the day, my mood, and who's asking.

From the snowcapped peaks of the north to the red-rock canyons of the south, Utah is awesome. I've visited places that I never imagined could exist, spanning five national parks, a half-dozen state parks, and nearly every section of seven national forests. All of these places—and the campgrounds within them—are so different, it's impossible to compare them, much less select just one as my favorite. When I started this book, I really did think I would be able to do that.

Instead, I've only come up with more questions: "What's in the East Tintic Mountain Range?" "How long would it take me to hike from Survey Lake to the Grandaddy Lake Basin?" With every trip, my to-do list has gotten longer instead of shorter.

In any case, the campgrounds in this book are the cream of the crop. Located in spectacular settings, each one possesses something special that lifts it above the average campground. Let your imagination and spirit of adventure see with fresh eyes, and maybe, just maybe, you'll be inspired to get outdoors a little more often.

In selecting the locations of these campsites, I've tried to balance easy access to some of Utah's best recreational opportunities with the ability to have a high-quality tent-camping experience. I've included, for example, incredible but lesser-known campgrounds that lie just outside most of the national parks rather than right in the thick of them. Exceptions to the rule are rare.

There are campgrounds near the big cities—Tanners Flat, Botts, and Snow Canyon State Park, among others—that will help you realize how truly fortunate we are in Utah to have immediate access to the outdoors, and there are more-remote campgrounds—like Clear Creek and Elkhorn—that will open your eyes to the magnitude of the outdoors at your disposal. Both kinds are a treasure and a delight.

Inevitably, fees get raised, campgrounds get renovated, and phone numbers and websites change, so visit jeffreysteadman.com for up-to-date information, including photos of each campground. You can also report updates you've discovered and help other campers (and myself!) stay informed.

So what's *your* favorite campground? Get in the car to chase the answer. There's so much to see, so many great locations, so many ways to enjoy each one. Who knows—within these pages, you might find a campground that becomes a family favorite or the perfect place to stage that new hike you've been aching to try.

I'll see you out there.

BEST
CAMPGROUNDS

BEST FOR SCENERY

BEST FOR PRIVACY

BEST FOR SPACIOUSNESS

BEST FOR QUIET

BEST FOR SECURITY

BEST FOR CLEANLINESS

BEST FOR WHEELCHAIRS

FAMILY-FRIENDLY

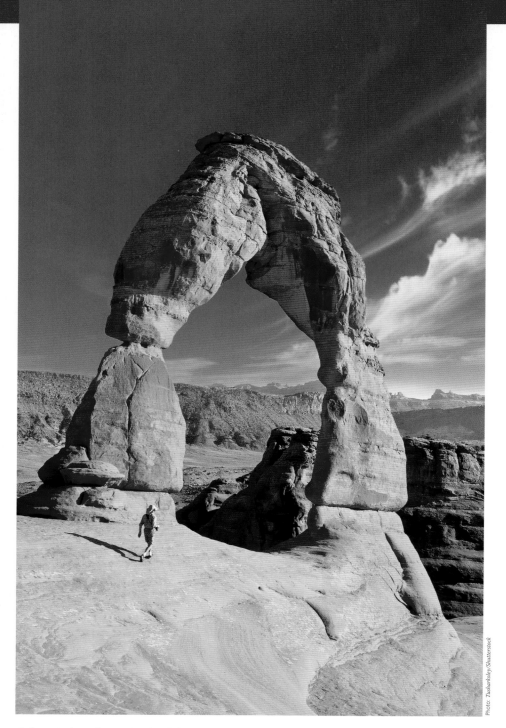

Delicate Arch, Arches National Park (see Hittle Bottom Campground, page 105).

INTRODUCTION

HOW TO USE THIS GUIDEBOOK

Menasha Ridge Press welcomes you to *Best Tent Camping: Utah.* Whether you're new to camping or you've been sleeping in your portable shelter over decades of outdoor adventures, please review the following information. It explains how we have worked with the author to organize this book and how you can make the best use of it.

Some text on the following pages applies to all books in the Best Tent Camping series. Where this isn't the case, such as in the descriptions of weather and wildlife, the author has provided information specific to the area covered in this particular book.

THE RATING SYSTEM

As with all books in the Best Tent Camping series, the author personally experienced more than 100 campgrounds and campsites to select the top 50 locations in Utah. Within that universe of 50 sites, the author then ranked each campground according to the six categories described below.

Each campground is superlative in its own way. For example, a site may be rated only one star in one category but perhaps five stars in another category. Our rating system allows you to choose your destination based on the attributes that are most important to you. Although these ratings are subjective, they're still excellent guidelines for finding the perfect camping experience for you and your companions.

Below and following we describe the criteria for each of the attributes in our five-star rating system:

★★★★★ The site is **ideal** in that category.

★★★★ The site is **exemplary** in that category.

★★★ The site is **very good** in that category.

★★ The site is **above average** in that category.

★ The site is **acceptable** in that category.

INDIVIDUAL RATINGS

Each campground description includes ratings for **beauty, site privacy, quiet, site spaciousness, security,** and **cleanliness;** each attribute is ranked from one to five stars, with five being the best. Yes, these ratings are subjective, but we've tried to select campgrounds that offer something for everyone.

BEAUTY

Exceptional scenery is practically a given throughout Utah, but five-star sites provide excellent views, and you'll know you're in a special place. The campground will be oriented to blend with and complement its natural surroundings, with the sounds and smells of nature rounding out the experience.

SITE PRIVACY

Ideally, trees, shrubs, and boulders or other natural features will have been left in place or incorporated into the site development to offer privacy and barriers between adjacent sites. The best campgrounds have well-spaced sites, with little visual contact between neighbors and a sense of solitude due to the campground's distance from the nearest roads and towns.

QUIET

Our top rating for quiet means you'll find little or no overhead or road noise, minimal social noise, an aura of solitude, and quiet hours enforced by staff (if there is any). It's a plus if you can hear the water from a nearby river or stream, the songs of birds, or the wind through the trees.

Admittedly, quiet is a difficult attribute to quantify because it can change quickly depending on your neighbors. In the case of this book, the author's evaluations were influenced to a great extent by the presence of RVs and the kinds of visitors a state or national park tends to get—campgrounds near urban areas, for example, are usually a bit noisy, as are those that cater to families with children.

The author also considered the extent to which you can get away from the fray at a particular campground. Expect some variation within the quiet rating based on whether you visit a campground during the week or on a weekend—on holiday weekends, all bets are off.

SITE SPACIOUSNESS

Spacious to us means plenty of room for two tents to be set back from the parking area and away from the fire ring. There should also be space for separate areas to cook, eat, and just kick back without being on top of your neighbors. The sites at some of these campgrounds are surprisingly large, even extravagantly so; others are quite small.

SECURITY

With a few exceptions, the author found Utah campgrounds to be very safe and secure, due largely to the presence of campground hosts and park rangers making the rounds. In general, campgrounds with hosts and those located where there is wireless coverage receive higher ratings than those without; we also check for an absence of vandalism.

CLEANLINESS

Everyone wants to see restrooms, fire pits, and picnic tables that are clean and a campground free of ground litter. If a campground is well managed—signs in good repair and up-to-date, buildings in good repair, and roads maintained—we give it high marks; things like noxious weeds growing out of control generally result in a lower rating. Also, while we take into account that primitive toilets tend to be a bit less tidy than modern facilities, we believe that there's little reason for either to be a mess.

THE CAMPGROUND PROFILE

Each profile contains a concise but informative narrative that describes the campground and individual sites. Readers get a sense not only of the property itself but also the recreational opportunities available nearby. This descriptive text is enhanced with three helpful sidebars: Ratings, Key Information, and Getting There (accurate driving directions that lead you to the campground from the nearest major roadway).

THE CAMPGROUND LOCATOR MAP AND MAP LEGEND

Use the Utah Campground Locator Map, opposite the Table of Contents on page xiv, to pinpoint the exact location of each campground. The campground's number also appears in the table of contents and on the profile's first page.

A map legend that details the symbols found on the campground-layout maps appears immediately following the Table of Contents, on page vii.

CAMPGROUND-LAYOUT MAPS

Each profile includes a detailed map detailing individual campsites, roads, facilities, and other key elements.

GPS CAMPGROUND-ENTRANCE COORDINATES

Readers can easily access all campgrounds in this book by using the directions given and the overview map, which shows at least one major road leading into the area. But for those who enjoy using GPS technology to navigate, the book includes coordinates for each campground's entrance in latitude and longitude, expressed in degrees and decimal minutes.

To convert GPS coordinates from degrees, minutes, and seconds to the above degrees–decimal minutes format, the seconds are divided by 60. For more on GPS technology, visit usgs.gov.

A *note of caution:* A dedicated GPS unit will easily guide you to any of these campgrounds, but users of smartphone mapping apps may find that cell service is often unavailable in the remote areas where many of these hideaways are located.

WEATHER

Nothing ruins a good camping trip faster than bad weather. Winter in northern Utah means that precious few campgrounds are even open. Southern Utah has more camping available in winter, but nights can still be frigid and the days drizzly.

Spring and fall are excellent times to visit the lowest and driest campgrounds in the state. Both provide excellent displays of nature's cycle of life: death and rebirth. Autumn is delayed into October and November in southern Utah, when giant cottonwoods along the small creeks light up in yellow hues. By March, the once-naked branches are slipping on their green leaves once again.

When the heat of summer settles in, campers flock to the mountains for relief. Snow remains in some campgrounds until June or even July, so check ahead to make sure that your campground has opened for the season. The weather changes rapidly above 7,000 feet in elevation; rain is quite common in the afternoon. Come prepared with ponchos, rainflies, and plenty of extra socks.

FIRST AID KIT

A useful first aid kit may contain more items than you might think necessary. These are just the basics. Prepackaged kits in waterproof bags (Atwater Carey and Adventure Medical make them) are available. As a preventive measure, take along sunscreen and bug spray. Even though quite a few items are listed here, they pack down into a small space:

- Ace bandages or Spenco joint wraps

- Adhesive bandages, such as Band-Aids

- Antibiotic ointment (Neosporin or the generic equivalent)

- Antiseptic or disinfectant, such as Betadine or hydrogen peroxide

- Aspirin, acetaminophen (Tylenol), or ibuprofen (Advil)

- Benadryl or the generic equivalent, diphenhydramine (in case of allergic reactions)

- Butterfly-closure bandages

- Comb and tweezers (for removing ticks from your skin)

- Epinephrine in a prefilled syringe (for severe allergic reactions to outdoor mishaps such as bee stings)

- Gauze (one roll and six 4-by-4-inch compress pads)

- LED flashlight or headlamp

- Matches or lighter

- Moist towelettes

- Moleskin/Spenco 2nd Skin

- Pocketknife or multipurpose tool

- Waterproof first aid tape

- Whistle (for signaling rescuers if you get lost or hurt)

ANIMAL AND PLANT HAZARDS

BEARS

The black bear is the only ursine species that calls Utah home. It's rare that you'll see one, although black bears inhabit the same areas as many campgrounds, especially in the mountains of northern Utah.

Take precautions in bear country by keeping your campsite clean and clear of food temptations, carrying pepper spray and knowing how to use it on the trail, and moving about in groups and not in silence. If you do encounter a bear, remain calm, but be ready to use your spray. Make yourself look larger than you are by raising your pack above your head.

MOUNTAIN LIONS

Stealthy and shy, the mountain lion is another predator you're unlikely to see despite its presence throughout Utah. Should you encounter a mountain lion that doesn't immediately retreat, stand your ground. As with bears, make yourself look large, stick with your group, and make noise. Don't run—that makes the mountain lion's natural hunting instincts kick in. If the cat attacks, *fight*.

MOSQUITOES

Culex mosquitoes, the primary type that can transmit West Nile virus to humans, usually thrive in heavily populated urban areas; in Utah, they're found everywhere from Salt Lake City (population 190,884) to Moab (population 5,046). They lay their eggs in stagnant water and can breed in water that has been standing for more than five days.

Although it happens only rarely, you can contract West Nile virus if you get bitten by an infected mosquito. Most people infected with West Nile have no symptoms of illness, but some may become ill, usually 3–15 days after being bitten.

Late spring marks the beginning of the heavy mosquito season in Utah. In the high-elevation forests, you'll hear the buzzing swarms before you see them. Their numbers wane after the first good frost, but you can find them in every season but winter. Protect yourself with an insect repellent that contains DEET as its active ingredient.

POISON IVY AND POISON OAK

You don't need to be on high alert for poison ivy or poison oak at most campgrounds in this book, but it never hurts to keep an eye out. In general, you're most likely to find the plants growing at lower elevations (6,500' or less) along rivers and streams.

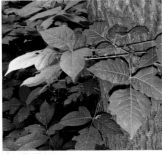

Poison ivy (*right*) ranges from a thick, tree-hugging vine to a shaded ground cover, 3 leaflets to a leaf; poison oak (*see next page*) occurs as either a vine or shrub, with 3 leaflets as well. Urushiol, the oil in the sap of these plants, is responsible for the rash. Usually within 12–14 hours of exposure (but sometimes much later), raised lines and/or blisters will appear, accompanied by

photo: *Tom Watson*

a terrible itch. Try not to scratch—dirty fingernails can cause sores to become infected, and in the best case you'll spread the rash to other parts of your body.

Wash the rash with cold water (hot water spreads the oil) and a mild soap or cleanser such as Tecnu, and dry it thoroughly, applying calamine lotion or a topical cortisone cream to help soothe the itch; if the rash is painful or blistering is severe, seek medical attention. Oil that gets on clothing, boots, and the like can keep spreading its misery for at least a year if you don't thoroughly clean it off, so wash everything that you think could have urushiol on it, including pets. In areas where poison ivy is known

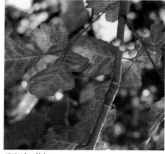
photo: Jane Huber

to grow, wear long pants and sleeves when practical, and keep your eyes peeled for those shiny green "leaves of three."

SNAKES

In my experience, snakes aren't a big concern for Utah campers—I never saw one while I was researching this book—although they may lurk in or near a few desert or foothill campgrounds. If you do encounter a snake, give it plenty of space and don't make any sudden movements.

TICKS

These pesky critters crawl up shrubs and grasses and wait for people or animals to come near where their outstretched legs can grab on. Hot summers seem to make their numbers explode, but you should be tick-aware all year round.

The ticks that light onto you will be very small, sometimes so tiny that you won't be able to spot them. Primarily of two varieties, deer ticks (which can carry Lyme disease) and dog ticks, both need a few hours of actual attachment before they can transmit any illness they may harbor, so the quicker you remove them the better. Ticks may settle in shoes, socks, or hats and may take several hours to actually latch on.

Wearing light-colored clothing makes ticks easier to spot, and an insect repellent with DEET helps keep them away; also visually check yourself a couple of times a day, especially if you've gone out for a walk in the woods. Use tweezers to remove ticks that have already attached—grab as close to the skin as possible, and firmly pull the tick loose without crushing it. Expect a bit of redness and itching for a few days around the bite site. If the redness spreads or you begin to experience fatigue or flulike symptoms, see a doctor right away.

TIPS FOR HAPPY CAMPERS

Few things are more disappointing than a bad camping trip—the good news is, it's really easy to have a great one. Here are a few things to consider as you prepare for your trip:

- **PLAN AHEAD.** Know your equipment, your ability, and the area where you'll be camping—and prepare accordingly. Be self-sufficient at all times; carry the necessary supplies for changes in weather or other conditions.

- **USE CARE WHEN TRAVELING.** Stay on designated roadways. Be respectful of private property and travel restrictions. Familiarize yourself with the area you'll be traveling in by picking up a map that shows land ownership. Such maps are typically available from U.S. Forest Service offices for a small fee.

- **RESERVE YOUR SITE IN ADVANCE** when that's an option, especially if it's a weekend or holiday or if the campground is extremely popular.

- **WHEN SELECTING A SITE, CONSIDER YOUR SPACE REQUIREMENTS AND MATCH THE SITE TO YOUR NEEDS.** Choose a single site if your group consists of 8 people or fewer, a double site for groups of up to 16 people, or a triple site for groups of up to 24. Group campsites in this book vary in capacity from about 16 to 100 people.

- **PLAY BY THE RULES.** If you're unhappy with the site you've selected, don't just grab a seemingly empty site that looks more appealing than yours—it could be reserved. Check with the campground host for other options.

- **PICK YOUR CAMPING BUDDIES WISELY.** Make sure that everyone is on the same page regarding expectations of difficulty (amenities or the lack thereof, physical exertion, and so on), sleeping arrangements, and food requirements.

- **DRESS FOR THE SEASON.** Educate yourself on the temperature highs and lows of the specific part of the state you plan to visit. It may be warm at night in the summer in your backyard, but up in the mountains it will be quite chilly.

- **PITCH YOUR TENT ON A LEVEL SURFACE,** preferably one covered with leaves, pine straw, or grass. Use a tarp or specially designed footprint to thwart ground moisture and to protect the tent floor. Before you pitch, do some site cleanup, such as picking up small rocks and sticks that can damage your tent floor and make sleep uncomfortable. If you have a separate rainfly but aren't sure you'll need it, keep it rolled up at the base of your tent in case it starts raining late at night.

- **CONSIDER PACKING A SLEEPING PAD IF THE GROUND MAKES YOU UNCOMFORTABLE.** A wide range of pads in varying sizes and thicknesses is sold at outdoor stores. Inflatable pads are also available; don't try to improvise with a home air mattress, which conducts heat away from the body and tends to deflate as you sleep.

- **DON'T HANG OR TIE CLOTHESLINES, HAMMOCKS, AND EQUIPMENT ON OR TO TREES.** Even if you see other campers doing this, be responsible and do your part to reduce damage to trees and shrubs.

- **IF YOU TEND TO USE THE BATHROOM MULTIPLE TIMES AT NIGHT, PLAN AHEAD.** Leaving a comfy sleeping bag and stumbling around in the dark to find a place to heed nature's call—be it a pit toilet, a full restroom, or just the woods—is no fun. Keep a flashlight and any other accoutrements you may need by the tent door, and know exactly where to head in the dark.

- **WHEN YOU CAMP AT A PRIMITIVE SITE, KNOW HOW TO GO.** Bringing large jugs of water and a portable toilet are the easiest and most environmentally friendly solutions. A variety of portable toilets are available from outdoor-supply catalogs; in a pinch, a 5-gallon bucket fitted with a toilet seat and lined with a heavy-duty plastic trash bag will work just as well. (Be sure to pack out the trash bag.)

  A second, less desirable method is to dig an 8-inch-deep cathole. It should be located at least 200 yards from campsites, trails, and water, in an inconspicuous location with as much undergrowth as possible. (Be creative and find spots with a great view—just make sure that you're not providing a great view for others!) Cover the hole with a thin layer of soil after each use, and *don't burn or bury your toilet paper*—pack it out in resealable plastic bags. If you plan to stay at the campsite for several days, dig a new hole each day, being careful to replace the topsoil over the hole from the day before.

  In addition to the plastic bags, your outdoor-toilet cache should include a garden trowel, toilet paper, and wet wipes. Select a trowel with a well-designed handle that can also double as a toilet paper dispenser.

- **IF YOU WON'T BE HIKING TO A PRIMITIVE CAMPSITE, DON'T SKIMP ON FOOD.** Plan tasty meals, and bring everything you'll need to prep, cook, eat, and clean up. That said, don't duplicate equipment such as cooking pots among the members of your group. Carry what you need, but don't turn the trip into a cross-country moving experience.

  On a related note, all of the campgrounds in this book allow responsible drinking on-site, but if you're visiting from another state, be aware that it's against Utah law to bring alcoholic beverages across state lines—if you get caught, you risk up to six months in jail and up to a $1,000 fine. Visitors should also be aware that the only adult beverage sold at Utah supermarkets and convenience stores is "near" beer (3.2% alcohol by weight). If you want to buy wine, "heavy" beer, or spirits, you'll have to go to a state liquor store (see abc.utah.gov/stores for a full list, including days and hours of operation).

- **KEEP A CLEAN KITCHEN AREA,** and avoid leaving food scraps on the ground both during and after your visit. Maintain a group trash bag, and be sure to secure it in your vehicle at night. Many sites have a pack-in/pack-out rule, and that means everything: no cheating by tossing orange peels, eggshells, or apple cores in the shrubs.

- **DO YOUR PART TO PREVENT BEARS FROM BECOMING CONDITIONED TO SEEKING HUMAN FOOD.** The constant search for food influences every aspect of a bear's life, so while camping in bear country, store food in your vehicle or in site-provided bearproof boxes. Keep food (including canned goods, soft drinks, and beer) and garbage secured, and don't take food with you into your tent. You'll also need to stow scented or flavored toiletries such as toothpaste and lip balm, as well as cooking grease and pet food. Common sense and adherence to the simple rules posted in the campgrounds will help keep you and the bears safe and healthy. (See page 5 for what to do if you encounter a bear.)

- **USE ESTABLISHED FIRE RINGS, AND BE AWARE OF CURRENT FIRE RESTRICTIONS.** Don't burn garbage in your campfire—trash often doesn't burn completely, and fire rings fill with burned litter over time. Make sure that your fire is totally extinguished whenever you leave the area. If you cook with a Dutch oven, use a fire pan and elevate it to avoid scorching or burning the ground.

  Note that bringing your own firewood from home is frowned upon by many campground operators, so check ahead to see if it's allowed. Bringing in wood from outside could introduce pests that are harmful to the forest, so if it's prohibited at the campground you plan to visit, use deadfall found near your campsite—again, only if permitted—or buy wood on-site if it's available.

- **DON'T WASH DISHES AND LAUNDRY OR BATHE IN STREAMS AND LAKES.** Food scraps can potentially harm fish, and even biodegradable dish soap can have a detrimental effect on fragile aquatic environments.

- **BE A GOOD NEIGHBOR.** Observe quiet hours, keep noise to a minimum, and keep your pets leashed and under control.

- **MOST OF ALL, LEAVE YOUR CAMP CLEANER THAN YOU FOUND IT.** Pick up all trash and microlitter in your site, including in your fire ring. Disperse leftover brush used for firewood.

VENTURING AWAY FROM THE CAMPGROUND

If you decide to go for a hike, bike, or other excursion off-site, here are some safety tips.

- **LET SOMEONE AT HOME OR AT CAMP KNOW WHERE YOU'LL BE GOING AND HOW LONG YOU EXPECT TO BE GONE.** Give that person a copy of your route, particularly if you're headed into an isolated area. Let him or her know when you return.

- **SIGN IN AND OUT OF ANY TRAIL REGISTERS PROVIDED.** Leave notes on trail conditions if space allows—that's your opportunity to alert others to any problems you encounter.

- **DON'T ASSUME THAT YOUR PHONE WILL WORK.** Reception may be spotty or nonexistent, especially on a trail embraced by towering trees or deep within canyon walls.

- **ALWAYS CARRY FOOD AND WATER, EVEN FOR A SHORT HIKE.** And bring more water than you think you'll need.

- **ASK QUESTIONS.** Public-land employees are on hand to help.

- **STAY ON DESIGNATED TRAILS.** Even on the most clearly marked trails, you usually reach a point where you have to stop and consider in which direction to head. If you become disoriented, don't panic. As soon as you think you may be off-track, stop, assess your current direction, and then retrace your steps to the point where you went astray. Using a map, compass, and/or GPS unit, and keeping in mind what you've passed thus far, reorient yourself and trust your judgment on which way to continue. If you become absolutely unsure of how to continue, return to your vehicle the way you came in. Should you become completely lost and have no idea how to find the trailhead, remaining in place along the trail and waiting for help is most often the best option for adults and always the best option for children.

- **CARRY A WHISTLE.** It could save your life if you get lost or injured.

- **BE ESPECIALLY CAREFUL WHEN CROSSING STREAMS.** Whether you're fording a stream or crossing on a log, make every step count. If you have any doubt about maintaining your balance on a log, ford the stream instead: use a trekking pole or stout stick for balance and *face upstream as you cross*. If a stream seems too deep to ford, turn back.

- **BE CAREFUL AT OVERLOOKS.** While these areas provide spectacular views, they're also potentially hazardous. Stay back from the edge of outcrops, and be absolutely sure of your footing.

- **STANDING DEAD TREES AND DAMAGED LIVING TREES POSE A SIGNIFICANT HAZARD TO HIKERS.** These trees may have loose or broken limbs that could fall at any time. While walking beneath trees, and when choosing a spot to rest or enjoy your snack, *look up.*

- **KNOW THE SYMPTOMS OF SUBNORMAL BODY TEMPERATURE, OR HYPOTHERMIA.** Shivering and forgetfulness are the two most common indicators of this stealthy killer. Hypothermia can occur at any elevation, even in the summer—especially if you're wearing lightweight cotton clothing. If symptoms develop, get to shelter, hot liquids, and dry clothes as soon as possible.

- **LIKEWISE, KNOW THE SYMPTOMS OF ABNORMALLY HIGH BODY TEMPERATURE, OR HYPERTHERMIA.** Here's how to recognize and handle three types of heat emergencies:

    Heat cramps in the legs and abdomen are accompanied by heavy sweating and feeling faint. Caused by excessive salt loss, these painful cramps must be treated by getting to a cool place and sipping water or an electrolyte solution (such as Gatorade).

    Dizziness, headache, irregular pulse, disorientation, and nausea are all symptoms of **heat exhaustion,** which occurs as blood vessels dilate and attempt to move heat from the inner body to the skin. Find a cool place, drink cool water, and get a friend to fan you.

    Heatstroke can cause convulsions, unconsciousness, and even death. If you should be sweating and you're not, that's the signature warning sign. Other symptoms include dilated pupils; dry, hot, flushed skin; a rapid pulse; high fever; and abnormal breathing. If you or a hiking partner is experiencing heatstroke, do whatever you can to cool down and get help.

- **MOST IMPORTANTLY, TAKE ALONG YOUR BRAIN.** Think before you act. Watch your step. Plan ahead.

NORTHERN UTAH

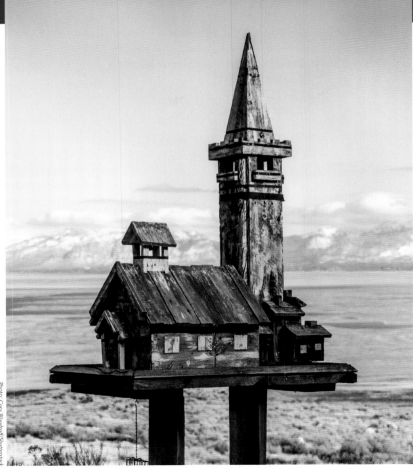

An elaborate bird feeder in Antelope Island State Park (see page 15)

⛺ Albion Basin Campground

Beauty: ★★★ / Privacy: ★★★★ / Quiet: ★★★ / Spaciousness: ★★★★ / Security: ★★ / Cleanliness: ★★★★

Albion Basin is where Mother Nature shows off her artistic side.

For a few short months each summer, Albion Basin operates as one of the quirkiest little canyon campgrounds around. A perfect example of the stark contrast between commercial development and land preservation, this campground has a charm all its own.

At 9,400 feet, Albion Basin Campground is probably the last campground in Utah to open each summer. The U.S. Forest Service simply lists the opening date as July, although the campground may not open until mid- or late July after especially severe winters. Call 801-466-6411 to confirm the exact opening date.

Albion Basin is a typical single-loop campground, but that's the only thing typical about it. You could say that the campground is located in downtown ski country, as it's bordered by the Alta Ski Area. The resort's Albion Lift passes directly over the campground, and in winter the campsites are visited by skiers on their way down the mountain. In the summer, however, the ski lift sits quietly above the campsites as a powerful reminder to take advantage of each day of summer; winter is always waiting around the corner.

Note: Albion Basin lies within Little Cottonwood Canyon, a protected watershed. Pets are prohibited here.

The campsites here are shielded well from each other, although I'd avoid sites 15 and 19. These two sites are set apart from other campers, but they're located next to private property with cabins well in view.

That trailhead marks the beginning of the Cecret Lake Trail. This 2-mile round-trip jaunt will take you up to around 10,000 feet, so be prepared to climb, especially in the last quarter mile. Don't be intimidated, though—it's common to see families with young kids making the hike. There's nothing more embarrassing than being passed by a 6-year-old on the trail, so

A Technicolor wildflower explosion in Albion Basin

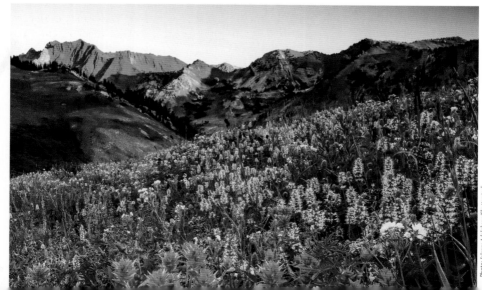

KEY INFORMATION

LOCATION: Albion Basin Road near Alta, UT 84092

CONTACTS: 801-733-2660, 801-466-6411, tinyurl.com/uwcnfcamping; reservations: 877-444-6777, recreation.gov

OPERATED BY: American Land & Leisure for Uinta-Wasatch-Cache National Forest, Salt Lake Ranger District

OPEN: July–September (depending on weather)

SITES: 25 (including 1 double and 1 triple)

EACH SITE: Picnic table, fire ring

ASSIGNMENT: First-come, first-served and by reservation

REGISTRATION: On-site self-registration or online

AMENITIES: Vault toilets, drinking water, garbage service

PARKING: At campsites and overflow lot at trailhead

FEES: $21/night (single), $42/night (double), $63/night (triple), $8/additional vehicle

WHEELCHAIR ACCESS: Restrooms only

ELEVATION: 9,400'

RESTRICTIONS:

PETS: Prohibited

FIRES: In fire rings only

ALCOHOL: Permitted

VEHICLES: Up to 25 feet

OTHER: 7-day stay limit; maximum 8 people/site (single), 16 people/site (double), or 24 people/site (triple); gates locked 10 p.m.–6 a.m.; off-road vehicles prohibited

keep your legs moving and you'll soon be at picturesque Cecret (sometimes spelled "Secret" on maps) Lake.

Despite its proximity to the town of Alta and its surrounding ski property, Albion Basin can take on a feeling of seclusion. Perhaps it's the immediate contrast of wild and domesticated land. Upon seeing the domesticated, you quickly identify yourself with the wild. It may be the small stream that wanders through the camp; its slow-moving waters create just enough background noise to blot out the occasional sound of a passing car or group of hikers. Still, it's a good idea to keep valuables out of sight, as there's a lot of day traffic coming in and out of camp.

Or perhaps it's the brilliant and hypnotic wildflowers that carpet the surrounding hills each summer. Who has time to look at a ski lift when there are showy blooms of wild geranium, penstemon, Indian paintbrush, and lupines in shades of purple, red, yellow, and white? The Albion Basin is where Mother Nature shows off her artistic side. There are hundreds of varieties of flowering plants in nearly every hue that delight visitors throughout July and August. Staying at the campground gives you a front-row seat.

If you're really excited about wildflowers, plan your camping trip around the Wasatch Wildflower Festival. This laid-back get-together of wildflower enthusiasts features hikes with naturalists who know the area. Some hikes start with a tram ride up the mountain from a local ski resort (Alta, Brighton, Snowbird, or Solitude). Live music and presentations help round out the event and make for a great reason to get away.

Albion Basin is also a popular place to start a mountain biking adventure. In the summer, the ski resorts offer miles of mountain bike trails. Forest Service trails may or may not be open to mountain bikes, so check with the information center about your plans.

Don't be put off by the 2.5-mile dirt road into the campground. It's well maintained and family-car friendly. It will be a bit dusty, but the dust won't bother you much at your campsite. Along the road, you'll notice a turnoff and parking area for the Catherine Pass Trail, which takes you up through Catherine Pass for a magnificent view of Catherine Lake. Here, you can press on toward the shores of Catherine Lake and farther to Lakes Mary and Martha, or you can continue climbing toward Sunset Peak. Numerous forks in the trail mean you can hike this area many times and always see something new. These forks also mean that investing in a good map will keep you from having an impromptu backcountry camping experience.

There are more remote and rugged campgrounds in Utah than Albion Basin, to be sure. But if you live in or near Salt Lake City, the convenience of setting up a tent high in Little Cottonwood Canyon, just 45 minutes from home, just can't be ignored—neither can the spectacular wildflowers and backyard hiking experiences. Ski lifts and encroaching cabins? Well, those *can* be ignored.

Albion Basin Campground

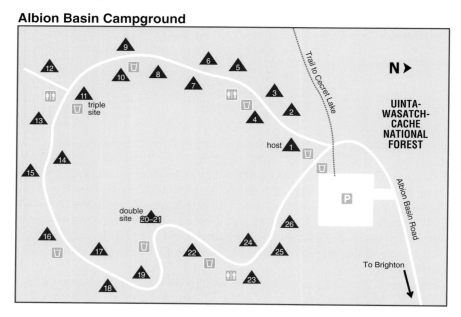

GETTING THERE

From the intersection of South 1300 East and UT 209 (East 9400 South) in Sandy, take UT 209 east 4.4 miles; then merge onto UT 210 (Little Cottonwood Canyon Road). Proceed east 8.5 miles up the canyon on UT 210; then bear left at the fork onto dirt Albion Basin Road, and drive another 2.5 miles to the campground parking area, on your left.

GPS COORDINATES: N40° 34.662' W111° 36.797'

Antelope Island State Park:
BRIDGER BAY CAMPGROUND

Beauty: ★★★★ / Privacy: ★★ / Quiet: ★★★★ / Spaciousness: ★★★ / Security: ★★★★★ / Cleanliness: ★★★★

From Native Americans to ranchers, the Great Salt Lake's biggest island has a fascinating story.

Northwest of Salt Lake City, Antelope Island is steeped in history. From Native Americans to ranchers, the Great Salt Lake's biggest island has a fascinating story. Stay at Bridger Bay Campground on the northwestern tip of the island, and you can experience firsthand all that this skinny island has to offer.

Evidence of Fremont people on Antelope Island pins their visits from 500 to 2,000 years ago, although archaeologists recently found a Humboldt-style arrowhead that could date back as far as 6,000 years. Modern settlement began here in 1848 when Fielding Garr moved to the island with his six children. The island became range for cattle, used to fund the Perpetual Emigration Fund (a revolving loan account that funded immigration to Utah for early church converts) of the Church of Jesus Christ of Latter-day Saints. Prominent citizens of early Utah, like Brigham Young, also kept their animals on the island. In 1875, the Mormon church gave up control of the island, and much of the property went to Union Pacific Railroad, homesteaders, and miners. Eventually land ownership consolidated into the Island Improvement Company, a corporate ranching enterprise that shifted ranching activities from cattle to sheep. In 1972, the island was sold to another ranching group. Nine years later, in 1981, the state of Utah purchased the island and converted it to a state park.

Antelope Island has two campgrounds. Neither is spectacular on its own merits; the setting is the selling point. Plus, telling your friends you spent the weekend camping on an island makes for a really cool story.

One of Antelope Island's resident buffalo

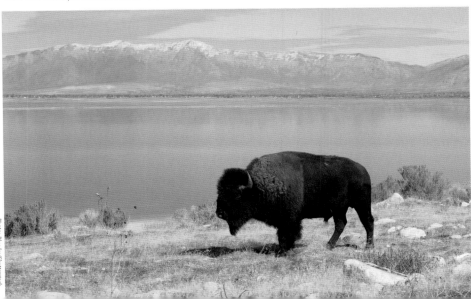

Photo: *Blue Ice/Shutterstock*

KEY INFORMATION

LOCATION: Bridger Bay Campground Road, Syracuse, UT 84075-6868

OPERATED BY: Antelope Island State Park

CONTACTS: 801-649-5742, stateparks.utah .gov/parks/antelope-island; reservations: 800-322-3770, reserveamerica.com

OPEN: Year-round

SITES: 26, plus 20 nearby group sites at White Rock Bay

EACH SITE: Picnic table, fire ring

ASSIGNMENT: First-come, first-served or by reservation

REGISTRATION: On-site self-registration or online

AMENITIES: Vault toilets, garbage service; drinking water, restrooms, and showers (except in winter) at Bridger Bay Beach

PARKING: At campsites only

FEES: $15 first night, $12/additional night, $13/additional vehicle

WHEELCHAIR ACCESS: Sites 20–22

ELEVATION: 4,260'

RESTRICTIONS:

PETS: On leash, at campsites only; prohibited at Bridger Bay Beach except for service animals

FIRES: In fire rings only

ALCOHOL: Permitted

VEHICLES: Up to 90 feet

OTHER: 14-day stay limit; maximum 8 people/site

Bridger Bay, the individual-use campground, has 26 sites, most of which are pull-through. While this campground attracts some RVs, rest assured that Antelope Island isn't the kind of place where you typically have to worry about raucous partiers. Instead, you'll find that most visitors here are fascinated by and respectful of the island's atmosphere.

The sites at Bridger Bay are spread around a large one-way loop. There's no vegetation taller than sagebrush, so you have to do without shade or shield from neighbors (hence the two stars for privacy). Each plot has ample space to pitch a tent on the grassy ground by the table.

White Rock Bay Campground, located around jutting Buffalo Point, is for group camping. You may want to check it out (especially site 1) if you're dead-set against staying close to other campers. The group sites are more spread out from each other, although the ground is only dirt and there's even less vegetation.

Antelope Island is heaven for birders. The Great Salt Lake supports between two million and five million shore birds—two-thirds of all migratory waterfowl in North America—and shelters one of the top 10 winter populations of bald eagles in the lower United States. Everything from avocets to white-faced ibis call this massive terminal basin home. If you're an avid birder, check out the Bear River Migratory Bird Refuge, on the lake's northeastern tip and accessed back on the mainland by going north on I-15 and then west on Bird Refuge Road at Brigham City.

You don't have to leave the island to see spectacular wildlife, though. And that's really the point of coming to stay at Bridger Bay: you've got wildlife all around you. In particular, you're sure to sight the common pasty-white biped (a.k.a. *Homo sapiens*) swimming in the Great Salt Lake. As a native Utahn, I take for granted the opportunity to test the unbelievable buoyancy of the salty (albeit stinky) water, but out-of-staters should try it at least once—it's a hoot! Staying at the campground gives you the perfect excuse; what's more, you have showers and sand about a mile away on a state-maintained beach.

Chase down more-desirable wildlife encounters by heading back toward the visitor center and then turning right toward Buffalo Point. Follow the signs to the buffalo pens to see some of the meanest-looking animals around. About 600 head of buffalo roam the island, so take the long road around the southeastern side of the island to historic Fielding Garr Ranch and you should see at least one buffalo in a more-natural setting. True to the song, the deer and the antelope play here, too, along with bighorn sheep and coyotes.

Fielding Garr Ranch has been preserved as a living museum, so take some time to walk the grounds and tour the different structures. The grounds are maintained by a caring staff; large cottonwoods dot the area to provide shade on an otherwise exposed landscape. It's a perfect place to plop down for lunch. You'll also appreciate the comforts of your own home after seeing the not-so-cushy living quarters of the ranch home. Take the time to read the in-depth description of the island's heritage, and you'll appreciate even more how special this place is.

Fall and spring are the best times to visit Antelope Island State Park. Even winter is preferable to the scorching heat in the summer. The bugs also kick into high gear when the temperatures rise, so plan to come here while it's still mild outside.

Antelope Island State Park: Bridger Bay Campground

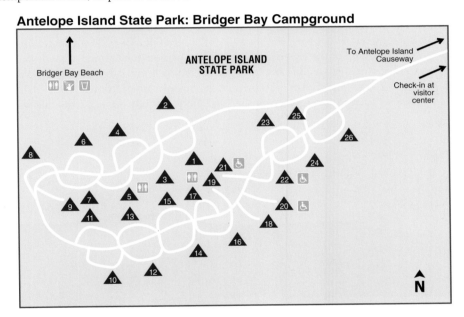

GETTING THERE

Antelope Island State Park is about 40 miles northwest of downtown Salt Lake City. From the intersection of West 500 South and North 500 West in Bountiful, with McDonald's on your left and KFC on your right, head north for 1 mile on North 500 West, and then merge onto I-15 North. Drive about 15 miles to Exit 332; then turn left (west) onto Antelope Drive in Syracuse. Continue west through town on Antelope Drive/West 1700 South and on across the causeway to the island, about 13.5 miles in all. Follow the signs to Bridger Bay Campground, which is about 2.7 miles southwest of the park entrance.

GPS COORDINATES: N41° 02.486' W111° 15.338'

⛺ Aspen Grove Campground

Beauty: ★★★★ / Privacy: ★★★ / Quiet: ★★★ / Spaciousness: ★★★ / Security: ★★★ / Cleanliness: ★★★★

This campground is where hopeful anglers begin their quest for the granddaddy.

Most people come to Aspen Grove Campground for one reason: to catch the big one. Sprawled out just a few hundred feet from the shores of Utah's busiest fishing water, Strawberry Reservoir, this campground is where hopeful anglers begin their quest for the granddaddy.

Not surprisingly, Aspen Grove Campground sits among a grove of aspen trees on the south side of the Soldier Creek arm of Strawberry Reservoir. The camp is divided between a squatty southern loop and an elongated northern line of campsites (think a balloon on a string)—53 sites in all. Not every site lives up to its billing as a shaded sanctuary. Here in the Uinta Basin, sagebrush rules the landscape; if a site isn't fortunate enough to have aspens, it's exposed to the wide-open landscape of scrubby silvered sage.

To be sure, there are RVs here, but it's a tale of two campgrounds. From sites 31 to 60, you're going to see a lot of the big vehicles, and they're packed in there pretty good, so definitely try to snag something in the loop, from 1 to 23. *Pro-tip:* If you can grab one of the three walk-in sites—12–14—you'll not only get privacy, shade, and a refuge from RVs, but you'll also be camped closer to Strawberry Reservoir than just about anybody else in a tent is allowed.

Strawberry Reservoir at sunset

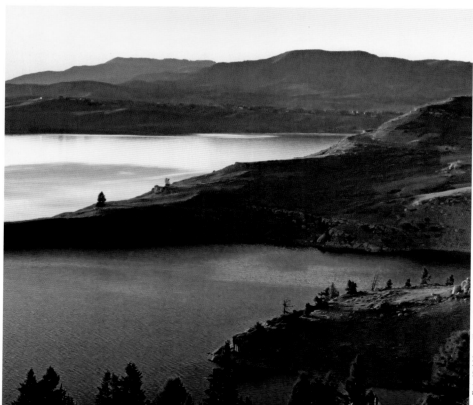

Photo: Mitch Johanson/Shutterstock

KEY INFORMATION

LOCATION: FR 482 south of FR 090, Heber City, UT 84032

CONTACTS: 435-654-0470, tinyurl.com /uwcnfcamping; reservations: 877-444-6777, recreation.gov

OPERATED BY: American Land & Leisure for Uinta-Wasatch-Cache National Forest, Heber-Kamas Ranger District

OPEN: May–September

SITES: 53 (includes 9 doubles and 3 walk-ins)

EACH SITE: Picnic table, fire ring

ASSIGNMENT: First-come, first-served and by reservation

REGISTRATION: On-site self-registration or online

FACILITIES: Flush toilets, drinking water, boat ramp, fish-cleaning station

PARKING: At campsites only

FEES: $20/night (single), $40/night (double), $8/extra vehicle; $8 boat ramp/parking fee

WHEELCHAIR ACCESS: Sites 33 and 34

ELEVATION: 7,670'

RESTRICTIONS:

PETS: Leashed

FIRES: In ring only

ALCOHOL: Permitted

VEHICLES: Up to 40 feet (60 feet for site 2)

OTHER: 7-day stay limit; 2-day minimum stay on weekends, 3-day minimum stay on holiday weekends; maximum 8 people/site (single) or 16 people/site (double)

If you decide to make reservations (probably a very wise idea on a weekend), take any site from 47 through 52 along the lower string. Venture above or below that magic range, and you'll be left treeless and out in the open. Also, don't go crazy looking for sites 24–30—they don't exist.

Strawberry Reservoir has an interesting past. It was originally built in 1922 as part of the Bureau of Reclamation's Central Utah Project, a boondoggle of water-development projects designed to bring water down to the Wasatch Front. In 1973, Strawberry Reservoir was enlarged with the construction of Soldier Creek Dam, and now the entire impoundment holds an impressive 1.1 million acre-feet of water—about 360.5 billion gallons.

Because of its size and location, the reservoir has always produced large rainbow and cutthroat trout. Unfortunately, nongame species like suckers and chubs have also flourished over the years. Special regulations, including the immediate release of all cutthroat between 15 and 22 inches, are in place to help keep the chubs in line. As a result, bigger and bigger fish are being caught from Strawberry. There are few other places in Utah one can go (Flaming Gorge, Lake Powell) to consistently catch such sizable fish.

During the summer, the fish go to deep waters. Shore fishermen may still find limited success in early morning, but float tubers and boaters net the most fish from about July through the beginning of September. Late fall finds the fish moving to shallower water, so October may be a good time to stay in Aspen Grove. Unfortunately, bad weather can close the campground before then, although there is some effort made to keep it open through hunting season, when the campground and surrounding area are very popular with the camo-and-blaze crowd. Call ahead to check the campground status.

Strawberry's absolute best fishing is had when the ice comes off the water in the spring. Again, the campground is almost certain to be closed at this point, but it's at least worth investigating.

Just a few hundred yards from the campground is a small boat ramp, complete with ample parking and a small fish-cleaning station. The ramp is considerably less crowded than the Strawberry Marina, on the reservoir's west side, so make a note if you have an aversion to large crowds.

Parents appreciate Aspen Grove campground for its family-friendly setup. Modern restrooms and the availability of drinking water make it a good choice for campers with young ones, and even the most impatient little angler can usually pull in a decent-size trout by floating a worm beneath a bobber at sunup.

If fishing isn't your thing, you may have come to the wrong place. The reservoir's south side is probably the best place to go exploring, but your immediate options are limited due to private property. Then again, if you're just content to be outdoors and you don't mind lounging around camp, the convenience of Aspen Grove will suit you just fine.

Aspen Grove Campground

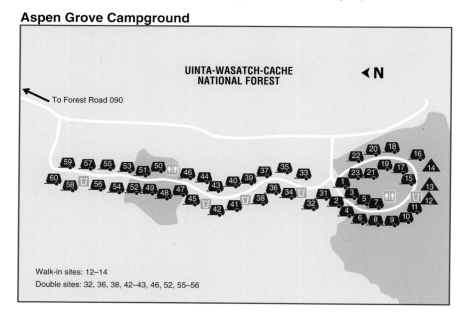

GETTING THERE

From the Y-intersection of US 40 (Victory Highway) and US 189 in Heber City, go southeast about 33 miles on US 40. Turn right onto Forest Road 090 toward Soldier Creek Dam, and continue 5.3 miles south to the campground entrance, on your left.

GPS COORDINATES: N40° 7.566' W111° 2.172'

4

Balsam Campground

Beauty: ★★★★ / Privacy: ★★★★ / Quiet: ★★★ / Spaciousness: ★★★ / Security: ★★★★ / Cleanliness: ★★★★

What Hobble Creek Canyon offers is a tranquil and serene setting for campers who love their solitude.

Not too many people could tell you where Hobble Creek is. Those who do would probably say, "Yeah, I golfed there." The next time you go up Hobble Creek Canyon, pass the links by, keep the clubs out of your car, and make room instead for a tent and sleeping bag. Balsam Campground is a superb place to camp.

Hobble Creek runs through a small canyon east of Springville—not the biggest creek or the biggest canyon. The campground is often passed over for consideration by campers who opt for the highest mountain, deepest lake, or lowest valley. Those campers can have their superlatives, though, because what Hobble Creek Canyon does offer is a tranquil and serene setting for campers who love their solitude.

The campsites at Balsam are spread out along the banks of Hobble Creek—some of which are accessible by footbridge only. That means tent camping reigns supreme here. Enter the camp from Canyon Drive, and you'll immediately see the group campsite to your right. A large parking lot and vault toilets sit on a small plateau above the river. Keep on the main road and pass the host to find the individual campsites.

Roadside view into Hobble Creek Canyon

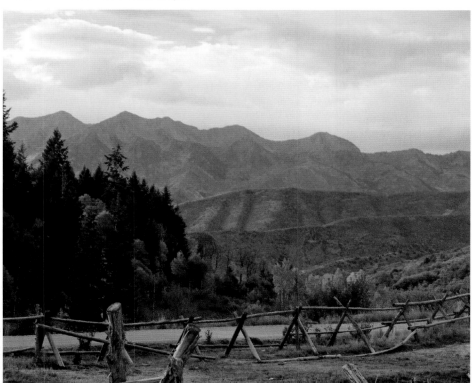

Photo: Dick Nielson

KEY INFORMATION

LOCATION: FR 058, Spanish Fork, UT 84660

CONTACTS: 801-798-3571, tinyurl.com
/uwcnfcamping; reservations: 877-444-
6777, recreation.gov

OPERATED BY: American Land & Leisure for
Uinta-Wasatch-Cache National Forest,
Spanish Fork Ranger District

OPEN: June–September (depending on
weather)

SITES: 24 (includes 14 walk-ins and 1 triple),
plus 1 group site

EACH SITE: Picnic table, fire ring

ASSIGNMENT: First-come, first-served and
by reservation

REGISTRATION: On-site self-registration
or online

AMENITIES: Vault toilets, drinking water

PARKING: Group lots

FEES: $20/night (single), $55/night (triple),
$190/night (group), $8/extra vehicle

WHEELCHAIR ACCESS: Sites 1–6, 10

ELEVATION: 6,000'

RESTRICTIONS:

PETS: On leash only

FIRES: In fire rings only

ALCOHOL: Permitted

VEHICLES: Up to 35 feet

OTHER: 16-day stay limit; maximum 8 people/
site (single), 24 people/site (triple), or 100
people/site (group); quiet hours 10 p.m.–
6 a.m.; off-road vehicles prohibited

After passing site 2 and the 100-person group site, you'll cross Hobble Creek on a little bridge and come to a small parking area. Through the woods behind the parking area is site 3, one of the most private in this campground. If site 6, the triple site, is unoccupied, site 3 is quiet and puts you close to the amenities; otherwise, groups at site 6 tend to expand the limits of the site until it reaches the edge of site 3.

Sites 13–16 are your safest bets for solitude. Park at the round parking lot at the end of the main road, and walk in to these tent-only sites. They're removed from the river, but it's worth the sacrifice to be tucked into the oak and maples in this section of the campground.

You'll notice that there are two footbridges alongside the camp road. Both lead to campsites across the river, but access to the first set (sites 17–24) is actually alongside the main canyon road in a large parking area. These sites are removed from the rest of camp, but unfortunately they're a little too close together and probably too close to the road for real comfort. The second set, sites 8 and 9, are a little more relaxed.

Pay attention to the road when you're finding your way to Balsam. After turning up 400 South, you'll come to a three-way stop sign—make sure you turn to the right toward the golf course. After passing the golf course, keep straight at the fork or you'll shoot by the canyon.

Hobble Creek has quietly become a favorite little spot for fly-fishermen looking to be driven mad. It's a small creek with a lot of underbrush and wary little trout. If you plan on fishing here, bring plenty of tippet and extra flies; you'll probably end up decorating a few trees with hand-tied dry fly ornaments. Sneak up on a fish, give the perfect presentation, watch him slurp your offering, and you'll definitely forget the frustration of losing a little gear.

You won't find many obvious hiking opportunities in the canyon, but the dedicated hiker will still find a few trails to explore. The main hike in the canyon begins at the trailhead where Wardsworth Creek enters Hobble Creek, just a minute up the road from Balsam. Take the trail for 3 miles along Wardsworth Creek to a small stock pond. Here, you can either turn around, joining the Dry Creek Canyon Trail to make a loop, or continue to Halls

Fork Road. If you take the trail to its end, you'll actually end up on the Great Western Trail near Twin Peaks and then Daniel's Summit in Wasatch County.

If you've got room in your car for both camping gear and golf clubs, throw them both in. Hobble Creek is a beautiful canyon golf course that runs parallel to the river and is flanked by tall trees on both sides, with stands of Gambel oak throughout.

After delivering you to Balsam Campground, the pavement ends and the dirt begins. If you've got the time, keep going and you'll reach the end of Hobble Creek Canyon and drop into Diamond Fork. The end of pavement also marks the end of camping-restricted areas, so if you're really fixed on the idea of being alone, pull off the dirt road somewhere for dispersed camping and all the solitude you could ever ask for.

Balsam has been flying under the radar for years, but I wouldn't count on that holding true indefinitely. Utah's ever-increasing population is constantly seeking new places to explore, and Hobble Creek Canyon just feels like one of those places that's on the cusp of being discovered.

Balsam Campground

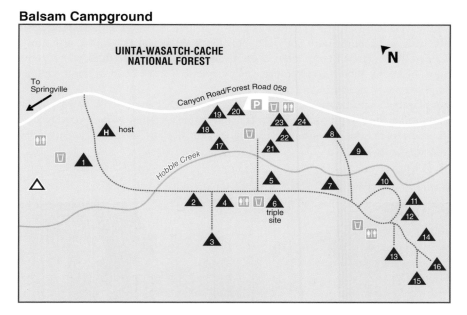

GETTING THERE

From the intersection of US 89 (South Main Street) and East 400 South in Springville, drive east on 400 South. In 1.2 miles, bear right around the traffic circle and take the first right onto Canyon Drive, heading southeast. In 5 miles, just past Hobble Creek Golf Course, the road forks—keep right (straight) at the Y to continue east on Canyon Road, which becomes Forest Road 058. In 6.7 miles, look for the turnoff to the campground on your right.

GPS COORDINATES: N40° 11.910' W111° 24.132'

5

⛺ Botts Campground

Beauty: ★★★★★ / Privacy: ★★★ / Quiet: ★★★ / Spaciousness: ★★★ / Security: ★★★ / Cleanliness: ★★★★★

The South Fork of the Ogden River is one of the best places to launch an inner tube and float lazily downstream.

East of Ogden on UT 39 is arguably the most concentrated clump of campgrounds in the state of Utah. Botts may be the smallest of them all, but it offers just as much high-quality camping as its big brothers nearby.

To reach Botts, you'll take UT 39. This two-lane road cuts through the narrow and winding Ogden Canyon area before opening up at Pineview Reservoir. As you pass the south shores of Pineview, take note of the campgrounds you pass—these park and picnic grounds suit large RVs and boaters, and as such they can become a little rowdy. Instead, keep going past Huntsville and leave the high-octane crowds behind. Soon you'll find yourself following the wide and rolling South Fork of the Ogden River as you snake your way slowly up the Ogden River Scenic Byway. Here, open meadows and immense trees exist together in seamless harmony. Before you know it, you'll come to a small bend in the road and find Botts—the second campground on your right.

For all intents and purposes, Botts and Magpie could be considered as a single campground profile: the camp host for Botts stays in Magpie, and that's where you register and pay for the sites at both campgrounds. Botts, however, has just seven sites and a more laidback atmosphere.

Botts campsite decked out in fall colors

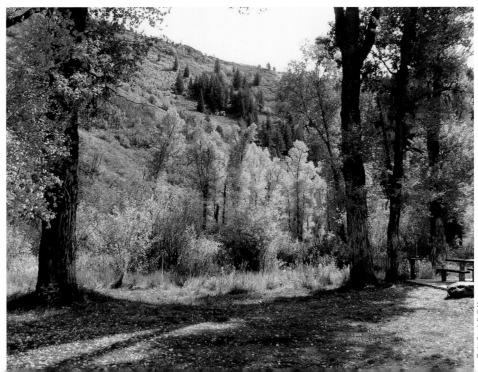

Photo: Beverly Duffield

KEY INFORMATION

LOCATION: FR 20078 just off UT 39, Ogden, UT 84401

CONTACT: 801-625-5112, tinyurl.com /uwcnfcamping

OPERATED BY: American Land & Leisure for Uinta-Wasatch-Cache National Forest, Ogden Ranger District

OPEN: Mid-May–October (depending on weather)

SITES: 7 (including 1 double)

EACH SITE: Picnic table, fire ring, grill stand

ASSIGNMENT: First-come, first-served; no reservations

REGISTRATION: Self-registration at nearby Magpie Campground

AMENITIES: Vault toilets, garbage service, drinking water

PARKING: At campsites only

FEES: $20/night (single), $40/night (double), $8/additional vehicle, $6 walk-in fee; $14 day-use fee

WHEELCHAIR ACCESS: Not designated

ELEVATION: 5,250'

RESTRICTIONS:

PETS: On leash only

FIRES: In rings only

ALCOHOL: Permitted

VEHICLES: Up to 25 feet

OTHER: 7-day stay limit; maximum 8 people/ site (single) or 16 people/site (double)

That's not to say that Botts doesn't have its problems. Because the river and the road are so close together, the campground is sandwiched between the two and is consequently a little closer to the road than is ideal. The South Fork does mute some of the traffic noise, but not all of it. Lock up your valuables to keep them out of sight to avoid being struck by a "smash and grab" criminal, just to be safe.

Each of the seven sites in the campground is immaculately kept. The main tables and campfire areas of each are cast in cement and are as neat as can be. Next to the cement area is where you'll put your tent. There are no actual tent pads, which is usually not a problem, but at Botts you'll probably have to get a little creative. Some sites have more obvious plots than others, though each is flat thanks to the topography of this river valley floor.

Botts is laid out like a curved needle, with restrooms and water in the middle of the small eye. Your best shot at staying away from your neighbor is in site 1, just off the highway to the right. Site 2 is also set slightly apart from the rest and is a bit farther from the road. Site 7 is detached from the others and close to the water and restrooms; on the downside, it backs up pretty close to the highway.

Staying here puts you in the middle of some prime fishing. Back down at Pineview, the reservoir flies in the face of the typical Utah trout fishery: while trout are present, warm-water species like bluegill, catfish, perch, and bass are more common targets. Pineview also boasts some of the biggest fish in the state with its healthy population of tiger muskie, a sterile hybrid cross between a muskellunge and a northern pike. These fierce fighters commonly reach more than 3 feet long in Pineview.

If the buzzing boats and suburban feel of Pineview aren't your style, continue up the highway to Causey Reservoir. Causey has no developed boat ramp and holds nice rainbow, splake, and tiger trout, as well as a few kokanee salmon. Try casting your rod near the inlets on either the Causey Estates or Boy Scout camp sides, but be cautious of current regulations. The inlets themselves are usually closed for large portions of the year.

You don't have to go anywhere for fishing, however, when you're staying at Botts. The South Fork of the Ogden River holds some nice trout, especially the browns. You may have to fight for space on the river, although not with other anglers—the South Fork is one of the best places to launch an inner tube and float lazily downstream.

Add an old inner tube to your list of camping essentials during the dog days of summer, and you'll be rewarded with one of the finest ways to spend a hot afternoon. Let the cool and slow-moving waters carry you downstream until you pop out of your tube and walk up to do it all again. Massive cottonwoods around Botts provide shade for an afternoon snack before you head back upstream to give it another run. (How long do they tell you to wait before swimming after you eat?)

When you're all through at Botts, say goodbye and resolve to come back up Ogden Canyon. There are enough campgrounds here that you could try a new one each time. Some are bigger. Some are farther from the road. But none have the unique charm of this little riverside campground.

Botts Campground

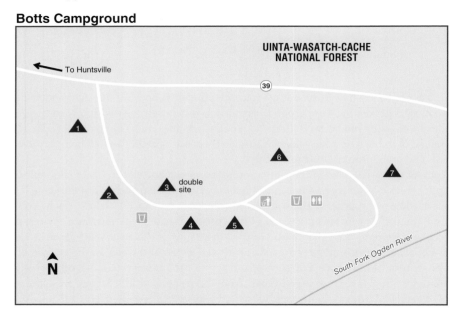

GETTING THERE

From the intersection of UT 204 (Wall Avenue) and UT 39 in Ogden, drive east on UT 39 to Huntsville. After about 12 miles, UT 39 curves north—about 1.2 miles after the curve, turn right onto East 100 South in Huntsville to continue another 6 miles on UT 39 to Botts Campground, on the right side of the road.

GPS COORDINATES: N41° 16.637' W111° 39.468'

6

Bountiful Peak Campground

Beauty: ★★★★★ / Privacy: ★★★★ / Quiet: ★★★ / Spaciousness: ★★★★ / Security: ★★★★ /
Cleanliness: ★★★★

Autumn drivers are treated to a canvas of magnificent brushstrokes of foliage.

A twisting road takes you higher and higher into Farmington Canyon on its way to a campground you'd never know was there unless you had already heard of it. On its way, it moves from dusty and dry surroundings with barely a tree taller than you, to scattered oak in a few clusters, and finally to a patchwork quilt of quaking aspen and evergreens. This is Bountiful Peak Campground.

Designed as one giant loop, Bountiful Peak has 33 individual campsites and 1 group site placed primarily among the aspen trees high in Farmington Canyon. The loop straddles a small hill, with the first dozen or so sites on the upside and the remaining sites down below.

Select your site carefully, because they're not all created equal. Try to avoid sites 6, 8, and 13—there are shadier and more-private sites to be had. Numbers 5, 9, and 12, for example, are probably among the best this campground offers. Site 14 backs up into a distinct bundle of aspens, and site 2 will require you to climb a few stairs to reach the table and fire area. The backside of the loop is where RVs have the best odds of parking, but they're not recommended at Bountiful Peak because Forest Road 007 is so narrow.

Precarious as it may be, you've got to love the road for what it offers in the view department. Early-summer drivers get to see a verdant landscape coming to life, while autumn

Bountiful Peak offers plenty of room to spread out.

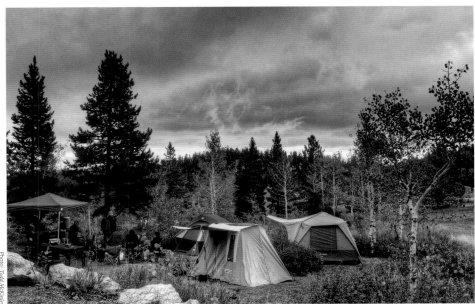

Photo: Todd McKinley

KEY INFORMATION

LOCATION: FR 007, Farmington, UT 84025

CONTACTS: 801-733-2660, tinyurl.com /uwcnfcamping; reservations: 877-444-6777, recreation.gov

OPERATED BY: American Land & Leisure for Uinta-Wasatch-Cache National Forest, Salt Lake Ranger District

OPEN: June–September

SITES: 33 (including 4 doubles), plus 1 group site

EACH SITE: Picnic table, fire ring

ASSIGNMENT: First-come, first-served; group site by reservation

REGISTRATION: On-site self-registration or online (group site)

AMENITIES: Vault toilets, drinking water

PARKING: At campsites only

FEES: $16/night (single), $32/night (double), $70/night (group), $8/additional vehicle

WHEELCHAIR ACCESS: Not designated

ELEVATION: 7,379'

RESTRICTIONS:

PETS: On leash only

FIRES: In rings only

ALCOHOL: Permitted

VEHICLES: Up to 24 feet

OTHER: 7-day stay limit; maximum 8 people/ site (single), 16 people/site (double), or 80 people/site (group)

drivers are treated to a canvas of magnificent brushstrokes of foliage. And in summer you can roll down the windows, rest your arm on the door, and feel the air becoming cooler and cooler as you make your way up into Uinta-Wasatch-Cache National Forest.

Because 100 East in Farmington is such an unassuming little road, you really wouldn't expect to be able to follow it to a tree-packed campground. Not too many people stumble upon Bountiful Peak by accident; in fact the only indication of anything interesting is a SCENIC BYWAY sign along Main Street that has nearly completely faded to white. Yet this campground has indeed been discovered. It has a full-time campground host—a rarity for a campground located so far away from pavement.

Despite its popularity and a lack of garbage service, the campground and adjacent areas stay pretty and clean. Know ahead of time, though, that everything you pack in, you've got to pack out. Plenty of people stay here every year and should be commended for their comprehension of that simple but sometimes elusive principle.

The summer months see plenty of campers traveling to Bountiful Peak, each for their own reasons. Some are Davis County residents who want a quick respite from the sometimes scorching summer heat. Others are families who make it a tradition to camp here every year. Yet others still find Bountiful Peak a more comfortable or at least more budget-friendly alternative to hotels or campgrounds around Lagoon, the local thrill-ride amusement park. Whatever the motivation, the campground offers a place for them all—or at least the first 34 parties to arrive. It isn't the quietest campground in the state, but it's a lot calmer than any other campground for miles around.

Once you've made the drive to the campground, you may just want to hunker down and relax. That's fine, but if you've still got some driving left in you, go back to Skyline Drive and take it all the way south until it dumps you out into the Salt Lake City suburb of Bountiful, a few blocks north of the Bountiful LDS temple. You'll get a spectacular overlook of Davis County right below Bountiful Peak. You might also try the Francis Peak Road route (Forest

Road 009) to the summit of Francis Peak. Things get a little dodgy toward the edge of the national-forest boundary, so pay close attention to posted signs for the latest information.

Children will appreciate the drive up to the campground. It's quite the setup for them to prepare for an outdoor adventure, and parents won't have to worry about water: there's plenty on tap, but none in the immediate area that would pose a hazard to wandering little feet. Even on a day trip, kids will be able to touch, smell, and see the outdoors.

Bountiful Peak Campground

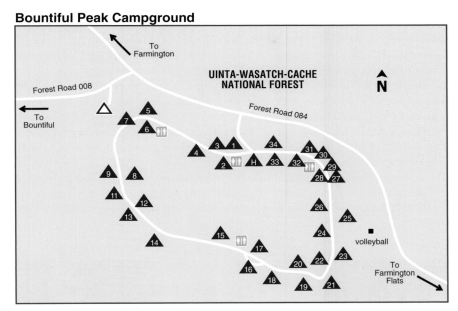

GETTING THERE

From the intersection of East State Street and North 100 East in Farmington, go north on 100 East for 0.9 mile; then bear right to continue east on Farmington Canyon Road, which becomes Skyline Drive (FR 007). In 7.7 miles, just after you cross Farmington Creek, the road forks—bear right to continue south on FR 007 and, in 0.6 mile, continue straight at a second intersection where FR 008 heads right. In another 0.1 mile, make a right into the campground.

GPS COORDINATES: N40° 58.840' W111° 48.274'

7

Butterfly Lake Campground

Beauty: ★★★★★ / Privacy: ★★★★ / Quiet: ★★★ / Spaciousness: ★★★★★ / Security: ★★★★ /
Cleanliness: ★★★★

The Uinta Mountains hold millions of adventures to be had by the willing camper.

Drive through the Uinta Mountains along Mirror Lake Highway (UT 150), and you may be tempted to stop at one of the many campsites before reaching Mirror Lake; there are 12. Do yourself a favor, though, and continue to lucky number 13: Butterfly Lake Campground. It's worth the extra few minutes on one of Utah's most breathtaking scenic byways.

Nestled against Butterfly Lake and tucked into towering pines, this road and single-loop campground has 20 sites, water, and vault restroom facilities. Arrive early and have your pick of meadow sites (14–16), lakefront sites (17–19), or more-secluded sites (1–3). The remaining sites are located around the loop in a typical wooded setting, although the healthy amount of space allotted to each is anything but typical for the Mirror Lake Highway area. Here you can spread out a bit and exhale.

From your campsite at Butterfly Lake, your biggest problem may be choosing which adventures to take. The Uintas are the only major mountain range in the contiguous United States that run east to west. With hundreds of rivers and small streams and more than a

Towering pines shelter this campsite.

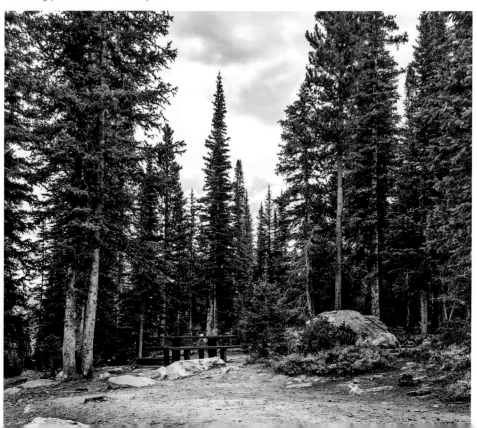

KEY INFORMATION

LOCATION: UT 150 (Mirror Lake Scenic Byway), Heber City, UT 84032

CONTACT: 435-654-0470, tinyurl.com/uwcnfcamping

OPERATED BY: American Land & Leisure for Uinta-Wasatch-Cache National Forest, Heber-Kamas Ranger District

OPEN: Memorial Day–Labor Day (depending on weather)

SITES: 20

EACH SITE: Picnic table, fire ring

ASSIGNMENT: First-come, first-served; no reservations

REGISTRATION: On-site self-registration

AMENITIES: Vault toilets, drinking water

PARKING: At campsites only

FEES: $18/night, $8/additional vehicle. A Mirror Lake Recreation Fee Area pass is also required: $6/3 days, $12/week, and $45/year; see tinyurl.com/mirrorlakepasses for buying information.

WHEELCHAIR ACCESS: Not designated

ELEVATION: 10,290'

RESTRICTIONS:

PETS: On leash only

FIRES: In fire rings only

ALCOHOL: Permitted

VEHICLES: Up to 30 feet

OTHER: 7-day stay limit; maximum 8 people/site; ATVs and motorized boats prohibited

---

thousand lakes dotting the map, these mountains hold millions of adventures to be had by the willing camper.

If hiking is on your agenda, then this campground makes an excellent point for launching off. For an easy, family-friendly hike, make your way to the Ruth Lake Trailhead about a mile farther down UT 150. The 1.5-mile round-trip trail is well marked and gains only 200 feet in elevation. Fishing and exploring are popular pastimes here.

If you want more of a challenge than Ruth Lake has to offer, make your way 8.5 miles back on UT 150 to the Crystal Lake Trailhead, just beyond the tightly packed RVs common at the Washington Lake Campground. Once at the Crystal Lake Trailhead, park and pick your poison. This trailhead hosts three separate hikes. For scenery, go with the hike to Island Lake along the Smith–Morehouse Trail. It's 3.5 miles each way and passes several lakes, meadows, and mountain views.

For even more impressive views of lakes dotting the entire mountain landscape, start on the trail to Crystal Lake and take the marked fork past Cliff, Petit, Linear, Watson, and Clyde Lakes. Another 10 lakes are within striking distance of Clyde.

Marjorie and Weir Lakes both hold arctic grayling. Though small, these feisty fish are a treat for the angler who has never caught one. Follow the Smith-Morehouse Trail over Mount Watson Pass, and then fork left at the trail marker.

For a more relaxing activity, try strolling around the southern tip of Mirror Lake on the boardwalk or picnicking back on Bald Mountain Pass. You're sure to have neighbors at both, but the views are worth it. Ten miles back from Butterfly Lake is Provo River Falls. Park in the designated turnoff and see the water cascade over staircases of slate. Bring a camera for sure!

Don't feel that you have to leave Butterfly Lake to take advantage of what the Uintas have to offer, though. Although fished frequently, Butterfly Lake still holds willing rainbow, tiger, and brook trout, and perhaps the occasional arctic grayling. It's stocked regularly, and the fish can be coaxed onto your line with small lures or classic worm rigs.

It's been said that being a weatherman in the Uintas is the easiest job in Utah; their line: "It will be gorgeous . . . until it's not." The weather can change unexpectedly, and brief afternoon rainstorms are the rule more than the exception. Come prepared and you'll welcome a few raindrops. Come *un*prepared and you'll find out just how many ways there are to say "damp." With an elevation of more than 10,000 feet, the area has winter snows that last until June or July, so call ahead to see if the highway and campgrounds are cleared and open.

Butterfly Lake is just 2 hours from Salt Lake City, so even here crowds can be an issue. Holidays, especially the Fourth of July and Labor Day, are extremely busy along the Mirror Lake Highway. Leave home early if you're planning to camp during one of those weekends. During other weekends and especially weekdays, however, you'll find this campground to be the perfect hideaway in the spectacular Uinta Mountains.

On you way home, stop at **Dick's,** a block past South Summit High School as you're headed back into Kamas on the edge of town (235 E. Center St.; 435-783-4312). It's open only seasonally, so don't be shy. Order a double bacon cheeseburger, fries, and a chocolate-banana shake for the perfect ending to your trip.

Butterfly Lake Campground

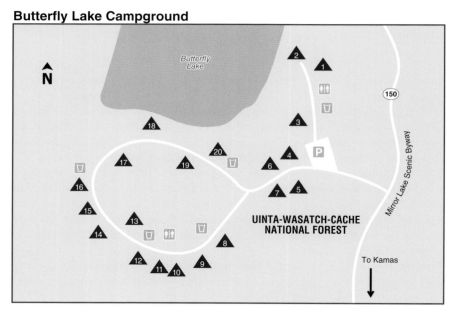

GETTING THERE

Take I-80 to Exit 155 (about 32 miles east of Salt Lake City and 42 miles west of the Utah–Wyoming state line), and drive south on UT 32 for 16 miles to the town of Kamas. Turn left at Center Street onto UT 150 (Mirror Lake Scenic Byway); continue east for 34 miles, and then turn left at the brown campground sign.

GPS COORDINATES: N40° 43.240' W110° 52.044'

8

Deep Creek Campground

Beauty: ★★★★ / Privacy: ★★★★ / Quiet: ★★★★ / Spaciousness: ★★★★ / Security: ★★★★ /
Cleanliness: ★★★

Deep Creek exists in its own little bubble.

Deep Creek Campground is one of those off-the-beaten-path campgrounds that make you question why you ever stick to *any* beaten path. In a region of Utah dominated by big and busy campgrounds in the Flaming Gorge National Recreation Area, Deep Creek exists in its own little bubble, just a few miles away on the north slope of the Uinta Mountains.

This serene little campground is a short string of sites with a small needle's-eye loop on the back side. Sites 1–4 are found at the campground entrance and offer two of the best sites in camp, 2 and 4. The campground road then passes a small bridge over the trickling waters of Deep Creek to the remaining 13 sites. Sites 5 and 10 will put you closest to the creek, but site 7 is where you're going to find the privacy and convenience of being separated from other campers and close (but not too close) to the bathroom. Site 11 backs up toward a large rock cliff and can give you excellent shade, for at least half the day.

Fishing is a popular pastime in this area, but hikers will find plenty to enjoy as well.

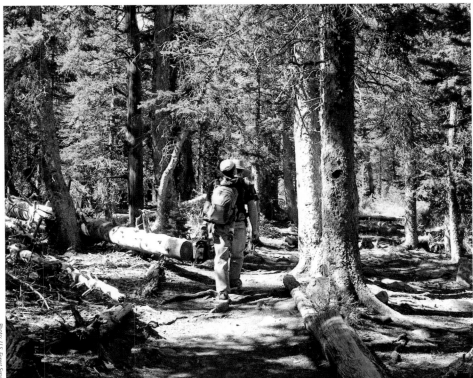

Photo: U.S. Forest Service

KEY INFORMATION

LOCATION: FR 539 west of UT 44,
Manila, UT 84046

CONTACT: 435-789-1181, tinyurl.com
/ashleynfcamping

OPERATED BY: American Land & Leisure
for Ashley National Forest, Flaming Gorge/
Vernal Ranger District

OPEN: June 15–September 15

SITES: 17

EACH SITE: Picnic table, fire ring

ASSIGNMENT: First-come, first-served;
no reservations

REGISTRATION: On-site self-registration

AMENITIES: Vault toilets

PARKING: At campsites only

FEE: $12/night

WHEELCHAIR ACCESS: Not designated

ELEVATION: 7,727'

RESTRICTIONS:

PETS: On leash only

FIRES: In fire rings only

ALCOHOL: Permitted

VEHICLES: Up to 30 feet

OTHER: 14-day stay limit; maximum
8 people/site

Aspen and Engelmann spruce form a patchwork of tree cover, while the waters of Deep Creek and frequent afternoon rainstorms provide plenty of precipitation for prolific brush, especially at the creek's edges. Be conscientious of the riparian habitat and the deadfall in the creek. Campers seeking firewood gutted the creek over time and unwittingly compromised much of the fish habitat, so the U.S. Forest Service placed logs and other deadfall back into the river to help restore it to health.

In fact, if there's one complaint to make Deep Creek, it's the obvious mistreatment it's had from campers over the years. A campground can't help but show wear, but it shouldn't have tear. Indeed, this campground is well used and will probably fill right up on the weekends, but its out-of-the-way location should only heighten the concern and care for such a nifty little place. Hopefully this renewed attention to the creek will help campers contemplate how special the campground really is.

Fishing opportunities abound in the Uintas, and this area is no exception. Deep Creek holds a few small rainbow trout, but for a few more rainbows, slide down to Carter Creek; located just past camp at the terminus of Deep Creek, it flows all the way into Flaming Gorge. Sheep Creek is also planted with rainbows—find it by continuing on Forest Road 539 to FR 218 (Sheep Creek Loop), or look for paved access on UT 44 back toward Manila, at the bottom of Sheep Creek Bay where it enters the reservoir.

High-mountain lakes dot the Uinta backcountry and almost guarantee the solitude seeker a chance at catching a pan-sized brook trout. Elk Park Trails 013 and 014 (you pass their trailhead on FR 539 on your way to the campground) will eventually lead to some of these opportunities, but in a very roundabout way. These trails are best suited for scenery seekers who won't be disappointed by broad views of Flaming Gorge. Alpine fishermen are better served by driving to Browne Lake or Spirit Lake on FR 221 and hiking anywhere from 1 to 8 miles for a choice of 30-plus little lakes.

Most visitors to this part of Daggett County come for the unparalleled fishing opportunities at Flaming Gorge Reservoir, more commonly referred to simply as "The Gorge." Monstrous lake trout have given rise to urban legends about dam repairmen refusing to dive without cages due to "car-sized fish." While those reports may be exaggerated, the current state-record 51-pound lake trout and 33-pound brown trout both came from The Gorge, so there are some brutes. The Green River is also touted as some of the West's best fly-fishing in the stretches just below the dam.

Within an hour's drive of Deep Creek you'll find no fewer than 25 campgrounds, picnic areas, or reservoir access points. This massive body of water and accompanying land area cover around 200,000 acres of designated recreational area, divided almost equally between Utah and Wyoming. While the reservoir has its unique and out-of-the-way campgrounds like Hideout Canyon (page 42) and another one on an island, most have one thing in common: they're usually packed from season's open to season's end. Choose to stay away from the madness. If you decide to go The Gorge, you'll just have to drive a few extra minutes from Deep Creek.

Truth be told, you'll find several sweet little campgrounds like this one throughout the Uintas. Deep Creek is one of the most accessible, and it serves as the perfect primer for what this fantastic mountain range has to offer. Do yourself a favor: avoid the crowds around Flaming Gorge, get off the main roads, and let Deep Creek Campground work its charm on your next camping trip to northeastern Utah.

Deep Creek Campground

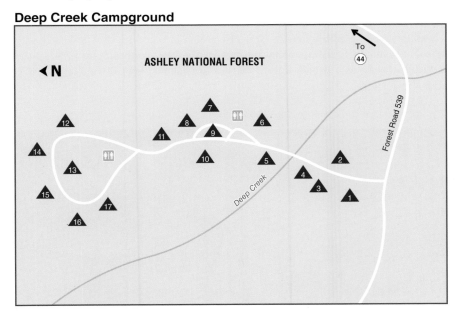

GETTING THERE

From the intersection of UT 44 and UT 43 in the town of Manila, drive 16.5 miles south on UT 44; then turn right onto FR 539 and drive 3.7 miles west to the campground entrance, on your right.

GPS COORDINATES: N40° 51.299' W109° 43.778'

9

⚕ Dry Canyon Campground

Beauty: ★★★ / Privacy: ★★★★ / Quiet: ★★★★ / Spaciousness: ★★★★ / Security: ★★★★ / Cleanliness: ★★★★

Something magical happens when people have to park and walk into a campsite.

The bridge over Diamond Fork at Dry Canyon Campground is bigger than necessary—the stream ripples but rarely splashes. Besides its obvious purpose as a means to cross the creek, the bridge serves another, perhaps more noble mission: it's the only way to access Dry Canyon Campground. All vehicles must park at the group lot just off of Diamond Fork Canyon's main road. Then, campers with their gear in hand (or on shoulder, strapped to back, or on head) must walk over the bridge and select their campsite.

It's only a few dozen paces, but something magical happens when people have to park and walk in to a campsite. "I wonder how long it will take us to restructure the accounting department" turns into "I wonder how long it will take me to burn this stick." It's miraculous. And it happens all the time at Dry Canyon.

Dry Canyon Campground lies about 10 miles up Diamond Fork Canyon, a smaller side rift in the larger and busier Spanish Fork Canyon, home to the reasonably busy US 89, which splits to send eastbounders to Green River and I-70 and southbounders all the way to Arizona. Diamond Fork Canyon's walls parallel the waters of Diamond Fork, a subdued little stream that flows downhill until it reaches the Spanish Fork River along US 89. The

At Dry Canyon, you get what you pay for—and so much more.

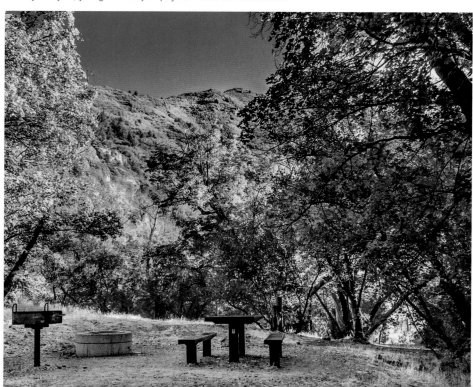

KEY INFORMATION

LOCATION: FR 029 east of US 89, Spanish Fork, UT 84660

CONTACT: 801-798-3571 (no website)

OPERATED BY: Uinta-Wasatch-Cache National Forest, Spanish Fork Ranger District

OPEN: May–October

SITES: 6

EACH SITE: Picnic table, fire ring, barbecue stand

ASSIGNMENT: First-come, first-served; no reservations

REGISTRATION: None

AMENITIES: Vault toilets

PARKING: Group lot; sites are accessed on a footbridge over Diamond Fork.

FEE: None

WHEELCHAIR ACCESS: Not designated

ELEVATION: 5,479'

RESTRICTIONS:

NONE OFFICIALLY, BUT USE COMMON SENSE: Leash your pets, be considerate of others, make fires in fire rings only, and don't press your luck by staying here longer than 14 days.

---

campground nestles in a shady section of the canyon, mostly oak trees, after the pavement ends and a well-maintained dirt road climbs to the upper segment.

Although the sites at Dry Canyon aren't numbered, I've put numbers on the map as an aid to identifying them. There are six sites in all, each one hugging the shores of Diamond Fork. The best hugger of the bunch, site 3, is closer to the level ground along the riverbed. Sites 1 and 2 sit away and up the hill just a hair, similar to site 6.

You'll have to get creative in sites 4–6 when it comes to putting up your tent. There's not a big opening of bare ground, and it's less level than you hope it might be. These sites do sit the farthest back from the road, however, so your creativity will be rewarded.

I'm just plain baffled about why there's no fee to camp at Dry Canyon. (The U.S. Forest Service doesn't even list it on their website, but it's there, I promise!) Sure, there's no water, but each site has a nice picnic table, a grill, and a concrete fire ring—amenities that could easily warrant charging a couple of bucks a night.

The most popular hike in the Diamond Fork Canyon begins at the Three Forks Trailhead, less than a mile away from Dry Canyon to the northeast. There are several trails to choose from, but the most well known is the Fifth Water Trail, which leads to the Fifth Water Hot Springs. These hot pools near a spectacular waterfall carry as much anticipation as they do precipitation. To find them, park at the trailhead and hike up the river for about a mile before crossing a bridge—*not* the first bridge you see near the trailhead. A good online search will give you detailed, step-by-step directions, so do your homework before you go.

Conservation projects over the last two decades have focused on removing nonnative fish species from the river and replacing them with Bonneville cutthroat trout. The resurgence of "Bonnies" in Diamond Fork began in 2006, and the fish are now protected from nonnative species by a barrier. Be gentle with the fish and the habitat.

Dry Canyon would be a camping bargain at twice the cost—heck, even 10 times!—and with any luck it'll stay that way.

Dry Canyon Campground

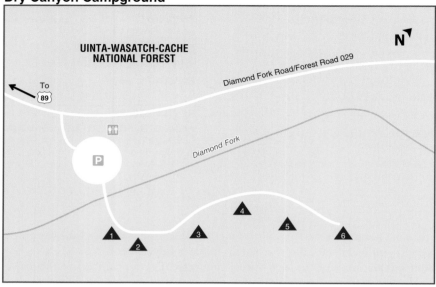

GETTING THERE

From the intersection of US 6 and US 89 in Spanish Fork, go 6.2 miles southeast on US 89, and turn left onto Forest Road 029 (Diamond Fork Road). Go 9 miles up the canyon to the campground, on your right.

GPS COORDINATES: N40° 4.782' W111° 21.846'

10

Forks of Huntington Campground

Beauty: ★★★★ / Privacy: ★★★ / Quiet: ★★★ / Spaciousness: ★★★ / Security: ★★★★ / Cleanliness: ★★★★

The air is always cool, the shade plentiful, and the camping unforgettable.

A chain of campsites dots the Left Fork of Huntington Creek just a few hundred feet from the spot where it enters the main creek. A small road leaves the main highway and drops down suddenly to the river's elevation, thick with heavy brush that drinks daily from the crystal-clear mountain river water at Forks of Huntington Campground. The air is always cool, the shade plentiful, and the camping unforgettable.

On any lesser creek, a campground at the fork of a tributary and its mother stream would be special, but on Huntington Creek it's really significant. Here, at just below 8,000 feet, two very prized trout streams combine their flows and create a dilemma for the serious fisherman: Which fork do I fish? In fact, the left, main, *and* right forks of the Huntington are all Blue Ribbon Fisheries.

There is a caveat, though. In 2012, the Seeley Fire ripped through the area for three weeks, destroying nearly 50,000 acres of vegetation. While the campground itself wasn't destroyed, the lack of vegetation upstream led to massive flooding all along the canyon, which affected many of the campsites here.

The campground was open only for day use until July 2016. Although the sites here still need some attention since the reopening, I have faith that the U.S. Forest Service will

The trailhead kiosk displays helpful information for campers, hikers, and anglers.

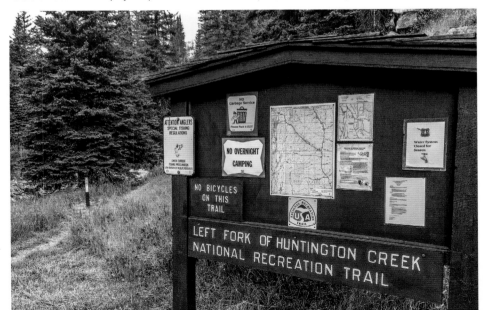

KEY INFORMATION

LOCATION: FR 0058 just off UT 31, Huntington, UT 84528

CONTACTS: 435-637-2817, tinyurl.com/mantilasalcamping; reservations: 877-444-6777, recreation.gov

OPERATED BY: Manti–La Sal National Forest, Ferron and Price Ranger Districts

OPEN: May–October

SITES: 5, plus 1 group site

EACH SITE: Picnic table, fire ring

ASSIGNMENT: First-come, first-served; group site by reservation

REGISTRATION: On-site self-registration or online (group site)

FACILITIES: Vault toilets

PARKING: At campsites only

FEES: $10/night (single), $40/night (group)

WHEELCHAIR ACCESS: Accessible restroom

ELEVATION: 7,600'

RESTRICTIONS:

PETS: On leash only

FIRES: In fire rings only

ALCOHOL: Permitted

VEHICLES: Up to 30 feet

OTHER: 14-day stay limit; maximum 8 people/site (single) or 40 people/site (group)

---

fully restore the best campground in Huntington Canyon, so I've included it in this edition. Should you find it not restored yet, head a few more miles up the highway to Old Folks Flat, where suitable sites exist.

Stay at Forks of Huntington while you're trying to devise a way to pick your favorite river, and you'll be in perfect striking distance of all three. You'll be plenty comfortable—especially if you came with friends. Site 1, a group site, will hold you and up to 49 of your nearest and dearest. Then the camp road rambles up the river to sites 2 and 3, which sit right next to each other and share a water spigot. Another trip up the road puts you at sites 4 and 5, also next-door neighbors. The camp road ends in a small loop with a restroom and the loner of the group, site 6. This is the most private of the sites when it comes to spacing, but it doesn't offer much cover from the road and visitors on their way to the restroom. Still, it's probably the site of choice.

With any lesser campground, a nearby hiking trail would be a great bonus, but at Forks of Huntington it's something to write home about. This isn't just *any* trail: it's the Left Fork of Huntington Canyon National Recreation Trail. A simple, connect-the-dots hike, it links Forks of Huntington Campground and Miller Flat Reservoir. The 4-mile stretch that starts at Forks of Huntington was designated as a National Recreation Trail in 1979, and for good reason. Scattered among the choice fishing pools are several small but scenic waterfalls. A simple snapshot of each one would make a wonderful wallpaper on your phone. Take your time behind the camera, and you could have a print that's worthy of a fancy frame.

There are other worthy trails in this part of Manti–La Sal National Forest. Go to the Stuart Visitor Information Center, a few miles farther up UT 31, to learn about such area hikes as Pole Canyon, Short Canyon, or a longer march through the Castle Valley Range.

An informational placard near the bathroom and parking area displays a map with high-lighted hiking trails and a chart that briefly describes each hike and ranks its difficulty. No matter which hike you choose, be prepared: the weather can turn cold quickly in these canyons, especially as winter approaches.

You may notice several small turnouts along UT 31. Some may indicate that an area is off-limits to camping, but most proudly proclaim THE FEE YOU PAY STAYS HERE and spells out a camping charge. These sites aren't anything glamorous—not much more than a scratch in the dirt, a fire ring, and no restrooms. However, they will suffice if Forks of Huntington is full. You'll miss the sounds of a river running by your tent, especially as traffic zips by on the highway, but you won't have any neighbors.

You've already got your fishing pole, so head to Huntington Reservoir, Cleveland Reservoir, or Electric Lake, all located along UT 31. They're excellent choices to get a taste of alpine fishing without having to hike in. Huntington kicks out some pretty beefy tiger trout and is a good choice for kids who want to cast from shore. Fishing conditions change throughout the year, but the go-to bait in these parts is a night crawler or minnow suspended beneath a clear bubble.

Forks of Huntington Campground

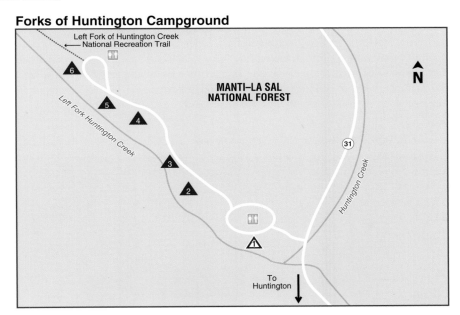

GETTING THERE

From the intersection of UT 31 and UT 10 in Huntington, travel northwest on UT 31 and, in 18 miles, turn left onto Forest Road 0058 to reach the campground.

GPS COORDINATES: N39° 30.036' W111° 9.468'

11

Hideout Canyon Boat-In Campground

Beauty: ★★★★ / Privacy: ★★★ / Quiet: ★★★★ / Spaciousness: ★★★ / Security: ★★★★★ / Cleanliness: ★★★★

If you've ever wanted to get away from it all—really away from it all . . .

If you've ever wanted to get away from it all—and I mean *really* get away—there may be no better place than Hideout Canyon. Although this campground is located on the shores of the very popular Flaming Gorge Reservoir, it might just be the perfect hideaway.

Should you choose to run away to this shoreline campground, you wouldn't be the first. Rumor has it that this canyon was used as a hideout by that notorious outlaw of the American West, Butch Cassidy, well before the days of Flaming Gorge National Recreation Area.

Technically, this 18-site campground is accessible on foot down a long dirt trail, and you can hike the 4 miles in. It would make for a great backpacking trip, as you have some amenities at camp, including running water and flush toilets, to reward your efforts. The trail is sometimes used by the equestrian crowd, but doing it on foot would make you one of the few brave souls on soles. Most people, however, boat in, then tie up and tent it out. In either case, you're guaranteed not to run into an RV. (The same holds true for nearby Kingfisher Island Campground, on an honest-to-goodness island accessible exclusively by boat.)

A "gorge-ous" view of Flaming Gorge Reservoir and Hideout Canyon from the Dowd Mountain Overlook

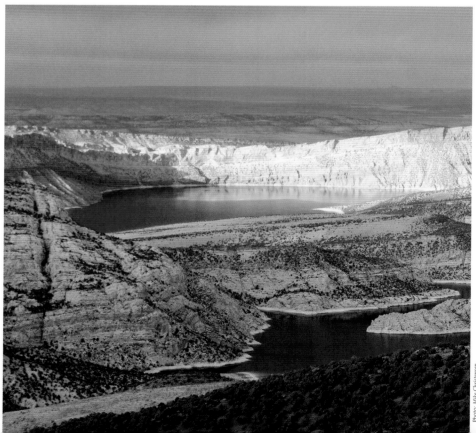

Photo: Mike Christensen

KEY INFORMATION

LOCATION: Flaming Gorge Reservoir, Vernal, UT 84078

OPERATED BY: American Land & Leisure for Ashley National Forest, Flaming Gorge/Vernal Ranger District

CONTACTS: 435-789-1181, tinyurl.com/ashleynfcamping; reservations: 877-444-6777, recreation.gov, or reserve america.com

OPEN: Mid-May–mid-September

SITES: 18

EACH SITE: Picnic table, shade awning, fire ring, tent pad

ASSIGNMENT: First-come, first-served or by reservation (recommended)

REGISTRATION: On-site self-registration or online

AMENITIES: Drinking water, flush and vault toilets

PARKING: At trailhead or boat launch; campground is accessible by foot or by boat only.

FEES: $22/night; boat-launch parking $5/day, $15/week, or $35/season

ELEVATION: 6,060'

WHEELCHAIR ACCESS: Not designated

RESTRICTIONS:

PETS: On leash only

FIRES: In fire rings only

ALCOHOL: Permitted

VEHICLES: Boats up to 36 feet

OTHER: 14-day stay limit; maximum 10 people/site

Once you've paddled, powerboated, or pumped your legs into camp, you'll reach your site. You won't want to arrive with your fingers crossed—and only four sites are currently first-come, first-served—so book up to four months in advance, up until the end of the season in mid-September. Each tent-only site has a picnic table with a small shade awning, a fire ring, and a tent pad. Flush toilets are open during the regular season; a vault toilet is available in the off-season.

While the remote location and limited access might have you feeling a little bit of almost-island fever, the limited tree cover still lets you know that you have neighbors. Sites are generously spaced; if you want to be away from the water, then site 6, 8, 12, or 14 will be your best bet. If you're the sort who wants to wake up and walk right down into the blue, then sites 3 and 9 will give you the most access. Keep in mind that the shoreline fluctuates from year to year and can even vary from month to month. Drought years will see more shoreline and longer walks to the docks.

The camp offers only sparse tree cover—hey, think of it as beach ambience. Utah isn't exactly rife with coastline, so close your eyes and walk through the sand thinking of breaking waves.

Don't keep them closed too long, though—there's plenty to see here. Should you decide to hike from camp, it's just over 4.5 miles each way, back up that dirt path. When you near Forest Road 094, look for a trail spur to the east, or just push on and take the road. Both lead you to the Dowd Mountain Picnic Area, where you'll be rewarded with sweeping views of Flaming Gorge all the way into Wyoming.

Flaming Gorge is full of adventure. Some campers choose to experience the region from a more forested point of view, and Deep Creek Campground (page 33) is perfect for that. Once you're at Hideout, however, you're probably not going anywhere unless you've boated in, and even then you're limited to the water. Good news for you: that water is full of fun times. From camp, you probably won't get a crack at the legendary mackinaw (lake trout) that inhabit the reservoir's deep waters, but the 91-mile-long impoundment of the Green River holds a bevy of other species: rainbow, brown, and tiger trout; smallmouth and largemouth bass; kokanee salmon; carp; channel catfish; and burbot.

Whether you get there by boat or by boot, Hideout is one of the most remote campgrounds in the state that still offer amenities like running water and flush toilets. In any case, you'll wake up not to the rumble of an RV generator but to the waters of Flaming Gorge lapping at the shore below you.

Hideout Canyon Boat-In Campground

GETTING THERE

Hideout is on the shore of Flaming Gorge Reservoir, about 20 miles south of the Utah–Wyoming state line. From the intersection of UT 44 and UT 43 in the town of Manila, drive 14 miles south on UT 44 and turn left (east) onto FR 094. Proceed 3.7 miles to the trailhead; then park your car and switchback 4 miles north to the campground.

To reach the campground by boat, follow UT 44 south from Manila as above, but after 8.1 miles, turn left onto FR 092 and follow it about 0.5 mile north to the Sheep Creek Boat Launch on Flaming Gorge Reservoir. Once you're on the water, navigate to the campground using the GPS coordinates below.

GPS COORDINATES: N40° 54.876' W109° 38.892'

12

High Creek Campground

Beauty: ★★★★ / Privacy: ★★★ / Quiet: ★★★★ / Spaciousness: ★★★★ / Security: ★★★★ / Cleanliness: ★★★★

This is one of those rare places that only the locals know about.

One word comes to mind when describing High Creek Campground: *rustic.* There really isn't much of a campground here, at least not a formal one. Two distinct sites do exist, but it's the allure of High Creek Canyon itself that makes this area worthy of consideration. This is one of those rare places that only the locals know about, partly because they don't like talking about it but mostly because they're the only ones within 50 miles of the campground, which is just 1.5 miles from the Utah–Idaho line and about the same distance to bustling Richmond, Utah, population 2,535.

These are all good things—very good things. They mean that the rustic sites at High Creek, and all the fun in High Creek Canyon, aren't in any immediate danger of being overrun with people. Sure, you might find the occasional Scout troop on a Friday night, or a large group at the Lions Grove (the local Lions Club's day-use area), but even if you find the two campsites already taken, you still have opportunities for dispersed camping along the road.

So why come to High Creek? What the locals don't want you to know is that it's a fantastic place to begin your exploration of the Bear River Mountain Range. Zippy little High

High Creek Lake, still wintry in July

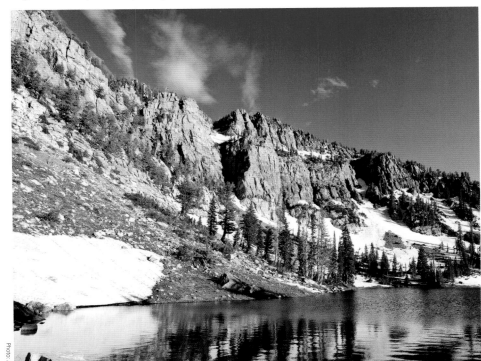

Photo: blog.ruffgurd.com

KEY INFORMATION

LOCATION: FR 048, Logan, UT 84321

CONTACT: 435-755-3620, tinyurl.com
/uwcnfcamping

OPERATED BY: Uinta-Wasatch-Cache
National Forest, Logan Ranger District

OPEN: May–September

SITES: 2

EACH SITE: Picnic table, fire ring

ASSIGNMENT: First-come, first-served;
no reservations

REGISTRATION: None

AMENITIES: Vault toilet

PARKING: At campsites or along the road

FEE: None

WHEELCHAIR ACCESS: Not designated

ELEVATION: 5,519'

RESTRICTIONS:

PETS: On leash only

FIRES: In fire rings only

ALCOHOL: Permitted

VEHICLES: No official length limit, but you
wouldn't bring an RV here.

OTHER: 7-day stay limit

Creek makes its way down the mountain, beginning just below the upper reaches of the range. At the peril of my own life, I will divulge that there are indeed fish in this river and they are, in fact, fun to catch.

High Creek also feeds the canyon with plenty of irrigation, so its shores are well shaded even in the lowest reaches. Segments of the creek are lined with cliffs, others with brush. Fishing isn't easy here, but for the persistent, the payoff can be surprisingly worthwhile.

High Creek flows right past the campground in some of its most accessible sections, so take advantage of the cool water. Even if used only for a few moments of contemplation, rivers are special things, and a campground with a river so close shouldn't be taken for granted. Both sites enjoy the shade of the canyon walls and trees along the river. The small vault toilet is tidy and well kept. The campground is just about the only sign of civilization in the entire canyon.

The road past the campground continues to a point where a four-wheel drive is probably recommended. After you can drive no more, a steep trail continues up the mountain into the Mount Naomi Wilderness Area and eventually leads you right past High Creek Lake on the Naomi Peak Trail, delivering you down to Tony Grove Lake (see Tony Grove Campground, page 85). The whole trek is 10 miles give or take, depending on how far up High Creek Canyon you trade in your tires for boot tread. It's a spectacular hike, rife with stream crossings, meadows, glorious views, and bright wildflowers at the right time of year. Just don't be disheartened by the fact that your entire day of hiking into the forest leads you to a parking lot at Tony Grove Lake.

When it comes to wildflower viewing, many people claim that the Bear River range is second to none. It isn't as accessible as some of the other contenders, so it probably doesn't get the same attention as places like the Albion Basin (see page 12), but the claim does deserve further investigation. Shucks, you'll just have to come and judge for yourself.

For an extended hike, take the fork of the trail that follows the north fork of the creek up Bear Canyon to the top of the mountain ridge, and you'll find yourself in Idaho at the crossroads of several different canyons. You'll just have to explore them all to pick your favorite— White Canyon, Boss Canyon, Deep Creek Canyon. They're all gorgeous and inviting. Use caution in these canyons, however, as they're all steep and can become hazardous, especially if there's any snow or rain. Check the weather ahead of time, and consider bringing a good set of hiking poles for extra stability.

Moose, elk, and deer wander the mountains in the Mount Naomi Wilderness Area, though they don't much make it down to the campground. Beavers are also abundant in many of the streams that amble down the local canyons.

You won't be swept off your feet by the elegance of the accommodations, but if you want a no-frills camping trip to an area where none of your friends have been, head up US 91 toward Richmond and into High Creek Canyon.

High Creek Campground

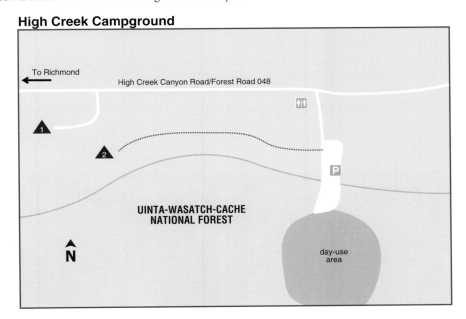

GETTING THERE

From the intersection of US 91 (North 200 West) and UT 142 (Main Street) in Richmond, head north on US 91 and, in 2 miles, turn right (east) onto High Creek Road, which is cosigned here as East 12100 North. In 0.8 mile, turn right at the intersection to continue east on High Creek Road, which is also variously signed as East 12300 North, East 12400 North, High Creek Canyon Road, and Forest Road 048. The campground is 4.2 miles ahead on your right.

GPS COORDINATES: N41° 58.586' W111° 44.110'

13

Hope Campground

Beauty: ★★★★ / Privacy: ★★★ / Quiet: ★★★★ / Spaciousness: ★★★ / Security: ★★★★ / Cleanliness: ★★★★

Stay at Hope and you can hop back to camp to change clothes, grab a bite to eat, swap your gear, and head back out to play.

If you're a local, it's hard to keep from giggling when you make the turn off US 189 toward Squaw Peak. Almost everyone in Utah County knows that Squaw Peak is where young couples go to spend "quality time" together. What no one seems to know, though, is that the road to Utah County's veritable Lover's Lane also takes you to one of Utah's best-kept camping secrets: Hope Campground.

Hope Campground is mere minutes from Provo and Orem, so you would expect it to be jam-packed with people looking for a quick weekend getaway—it's the only overnight campground located in the immediate Provo Canyon area, after all. How delightful, then, to discover you've got a good chance at finding a vacancy among the 24 sites here, even on

Bridal Veil Falls in Provo Canyon

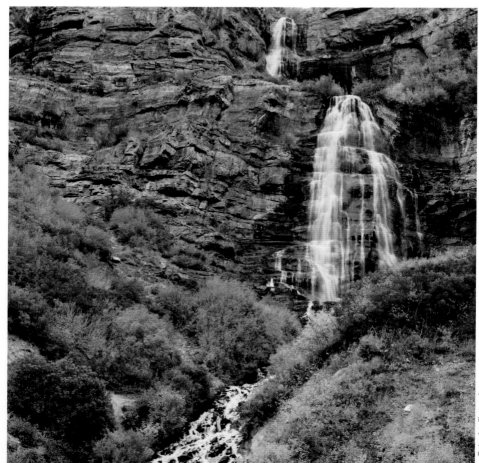

Photo: *alysta/Shutterstock*

KEY INFORMATION

LOCATION: Squaw Peak Road (FR 027), Provo, UT 84604

CONTACTS: 801-785-3563, tinyurl.com/uwcnfcamping; reservations: 877-444-6677, recreation.gov

OPERATED BY: American Land & Leisure for Uinta-Wasatch-Cache National Forest, Pleasant Grove Ranger District

OPEN: Late May–October (depending on weather)

SITES: 24 (including 2 doubles)

EACH SITE: Picnic table, fire ring, barbecue stand

ASSIGNMENT: First-come, first-served and by reservation

REGISTRATION: On-site self-registration or online

AMENITIES: Vault toilets

PARKING: At campsites only

FEES: $21/night (single), $42/night (double), $8/extra vehicle; $8 day-use fee

WHEELCHAIR ACCESS: Not designated

ELEVATION: 6,660'

RESTRICTIONS:

PETS: On leash only

FIRES: In fire rings only

ALCOHOL: Permitted

VEHICLES: Up to 35 feet

OTHER: 7-day stay limit; maximum 8 people/site (single) or 16 people/site (double); gates locked 10 p.m.–7 a.m.; off-road vehicles and horses prohibited; bring your own drinking water

---

a weekend. Also, the road forks below the campground, sending sweethearts one way and serious campers the other.

With a name like Hope, the campground may tempt you to run up the canyon and look for an empty site. Although it's likely that you could do just that, you should still probably try to book ahead of time. Family reunions or large group activities can fill this camp quickly—better safe than sorry.

After leaving the pavement above the campground, you'll descend on a dirt road to find the sites. Hope is a long, oval loop cut down the middle with another straight road. Campsites line the outer loop on both sides of the road as well as both sides of the bisecting road. The sites here sit under a shady mixture of oak and a few maple trees. At 6,600 feet, you're not quite in pine tree territory, so you definitely don't get a high-mountain feel, especially during sizzling daytime hours.

You won't enjoy extreme privacy at Hope, but you won't feel like your personal space is constantly being invaded either. Site 3 is above the road to the left as you first enter and would allow you to hide your tent away quite nicely. Park at site 8, and you'll climb a few stairs and disappear behind some of the low-growing vegetation. Conversely, site 5 is right on the road and would make you feel that you could be run over at any minute while sitting in your tent.

Provo Canyon is a popular place for many different reasons. Families flock to the area for its many parks and places to picnic and play. Teens and college kids come to float the Provo River in inner tubes and, inevitably, have a water fight. Anglers are in love with the Provo River for the big browns and rainbows it's been known to churn out. It's Utah's most popular stretch of river, deserving every bit of its Blue Ribbon status. Paddlers get in on the action for the long, smooth beginner rides in several stretches in the canyon. The Provo River Parkway Trail, a paved walkway along the shores, draws inline skaters, bikers, and exercise enthusiasts looking for a change of pace.

Stay at Hope and you can hop back to camp to change clothes, grab a bite to eat, swap your gear, and head back out to play. Just be mindful of private-property lines along the canyon, as there are quite a few. When in doubt, stick to the specially marked public-access areas.

Be sure to visit Bridal Veil Falls, just up the canyon from Squaw Peak Road along US 189. This spectacular 607-foot waterfall cascades over layers of rock on its way to a small and enchanting pool along the canyon floor. Drive right to the pool area and kink your neck trying to follow a single drop as it twists, turns, crashes, and tumbles its way down. You'll also see the remains of a tramway that once held the distinctive honor of being the world's steepest tram—now out of operation due to avalanche damage in 1997.

If you were to ask the typical Squaw Peak visitor what's at the end of Squaw Peak Road, more than one would probably say "hope" of the romantic kind. Little do they (and most others) know that's the name of an inviting little campground just minutes from the noise of Utah County.

Hope Campground

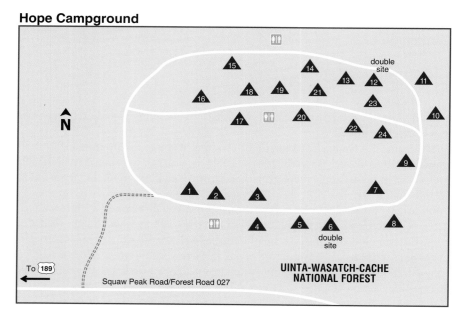

GETTING THERE

From the junction of UT 52 (800 North) and US 189 in Orem, take US 189 east up Provo Canyon. In 2 miles, turn right (south) onto Squaw Peak Road (Forest Road 027); in 4.5 miles, make a left at the signed turnoff and drive another 0.3 mile to the campground. (The campground sign is small and easy to miss if you're not paying attention.)

GPS COORDINATES: N40° 18.282' W111° 37.158'

14

Jordanelle State Park:
ROCK CLIFF CAMPGROUND

Beauty: ★★★★★ / Privacy: ★★★ / Quiet: ★★★★ / Spaciousness: ★★★★ / Security: ★★★★ /
Cleanliness: ★★★★

Leave your tent and you'll be angling at Utah's best fishing river in less than 60 seconds.

From its headwaters high in the Uinta Mountains, down a rocky, timbered riverway through narrow cascading canyons, with sinuous stretches among the meadows, the Provo River is a waterway of constant change. In 1993, the river was changed dramatically when a dam was built near Heber City to capture water for growing municipal and industrial use by the burgeoning populations below. The result is the 320,000 acre-foot Jordanelle Reservoir and, as a by-product, Jordanelle State Park.

The park has two distinct camping areas. The larger and louder is the huge Hailstone complex, which hosts a marina, boat launch, restaurant, and day-use area with pavilions, beaches, and a playground. The colossal recreation complex on the western shore of the reservoir also holds 10 distinct camping areas, with 28 sites on the Keetley Loop appointed just for tenters.

Skip the madness and constant commotion that define Hailstone and drive around to the Rock Cliff Campground, on Jordanelle's southeastern shore. Utah State Parks got it right here, creating a more tranquil alternative to Hailstone. All four areas at Rock Cliff—Rock View, Upland Meadow, Aspen Grove, and Riverbend—comprise walk-in tent sites near the banks of the Provo River as it enters the reservoir. Park in one of the group parking lots and haul your gear over the boardwalks spanning the marshes below, and you can choose from 48 different sites tailored to a tenter's needs.

Fed by the Provo River, Jordanelle Reservoir helps provide drinking water for a three-county area.

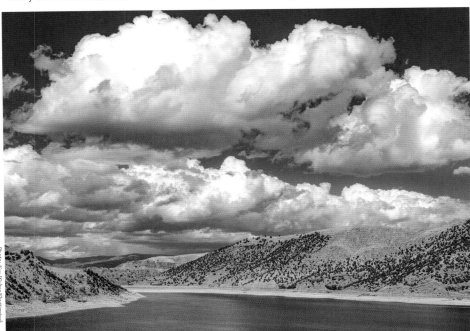

Photo: Ken Wolter/Shutterstock

KEY INFORMATION

LOCATION: UT 319 east of US 40, Heber City, UT 84032

CONTACTS: 435-649-9540, stateparks.utah.gov/parks/jordanelle; reservations: 800-322-3770, reserveamerica.com

OPERATED BY: Jordanelle State Park

OPEN: May 15–September 30

SITES: 48 (walk-in), plus 1 group site

EACH SITE: Picnic table, tent pad, fire ring

ASSIGNMENT: First-come, first-served and by reservation Memorial Day–Labor Day

REGISTRATION: On-site self-registration or online

AMENITIES: Flush toilets, showers, drinking water, fish-cleaning stations, nature center, small boat launch

PARKING: In group lots only

FEES: $20/night, $10/additional vehicle; $7 day-use fee. See park website for additional fees by season and facility.

ELEVATION: 6,150'

WHEELCHAIR ACCESS: Rock View sites 1–3

RESTRICTIONS:

PETS: Prohibited in Rock Cliff but permitted in other parts of the park. See park website for specifics.

FIRES: In fire rings only

ALCOHOL: Permitted

VEHICLES: N/A

OTHER: 14-day stay limit; maximum 8 people, 1 tent/site

At 6,150 feet, this campground isn't exactly up in the alpine air, so the shade provided by the enormous riparian corridor cottonwoods is something to cherish. At Hailstone, they just don't have this luxury. Rock View (sites 1–7) was built to meet ADA standards and is closest to the parking areas on the near side of the river. Reach Riverbend (sites 8–16), Aspen Grove (sites 17–36), and Upland Meadow (sites 37–51) by crossing the Provo River over a footbridge. Each site is clean and neat, spread out among the crisscrossing footpaths.

Booking a site at Rock Cliff online can be confusing. Be sure to select "Rock Cliff" when searching reserveamerica.com—searching for just "Jordanelle" pulls up the sites at Hailstone, and it's hard to navigate to the Rock Cliff side. Reservations are accepted Memorial Day–Labor Day, but your chances of getting a site by simply showing up are actually quite good, save for busy weekends and holidays.

Fishermen love the Provo River. It's the single-most fished river in the state, and with good reason. Here, where it enters Jordanelle, you'll find a good mix of rainbow and brown trout. Rock Cliff will make you feel like you're in a fishing camp of yesteryear—the kind where men wore flannel plaid shirts and had long, bushy beards. Flannel-clad or not, leave your tent and you'll be angling at Utah's best fishing river in less than 60 seconds. Try throwing a small silver spinner upstream and zipping it back as fast as you can. Depending on the time of year, a bead-head prince nymph flung by a fly rod can catch the attention of cruising beasts.

The reservoir itself offers more family-friendly fishing. Standard baits seem to always produce a good rainbow trout or two, sometimes many more depending on the day. In addition, bass fishermen are now falling in love with Jordanelle for its recent ability to produce some beefy smallmouth. Check the current *Utah Fishing Guidebook* (available as a free download at wildlife.utah.gov/utah-fishing-guidebook.html) or wildlife.utah.gov/hotspots for the latest information about the area; both the reservoir and the river have special regulations and are closely monitored.

If fishing isn't your thing, fear not. Mosey on in to the nature center by the campground to learn more about the fragile wetland area around Rock Cliff and some of the creatures that call the area home. The nature center offers presentations in its theater nearly every day and campfire programs to help visitors deepen their appreciation for this special place.

Birders flock (pun intended) to Rock Cliff to see such species as golden eagles, red-tailed hawks, and the nocturnal great horned owl that live in or visit in the region. The wetlands also host a bevy of big game including mule deer, elk, and moose. I visited on a weekday just after the campground had opened for the summer, and as I rounded a corner near the nature center, I found myself face to face with a big mama moose—only 15 feet away! After catching my breath, I got a great photo of the big beast and backed away slowly. (I was later grateful for Rock Cliff's tidy restrooms.)

With so much nature to see and experience in and around Rock Cliff, you'll hardly have a reason to leave. While it's sad to see this section of the wild Provo River now tamed, it has created new kinds of recreation and a terrific place to camp.

Jordanelle State Park: Rock Cliff Campground

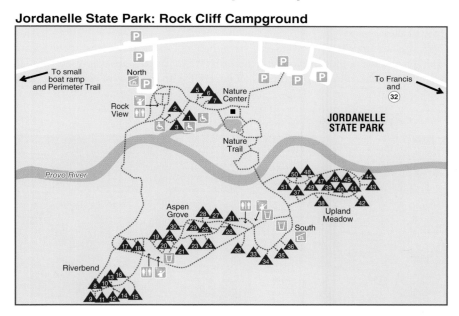

GETTING THERE

From the intersection of UT 32 and UT 35 in the town of Francis, drive 3.1 miles west on UT 32, and then turn right onto the campground entrance road.

GPS COORDINATES: N40° 36.283' W111° 20.309'

15

Lodge Campground

Beauty: ★★★★ / Privacy: ★★★ / Quiet: ★★★ / Spaciousness: ★★★ / Security: ★★★★ / Cleanliness: ★★★★

Lodge Campground has about 10 big brothers and sisters scattered throughout Logan Canyon. It's this status—as the runt of the litter—that makes it a unique and charming little place for tenters to enjoy.

You'll find Lodge Campground off US 89 just east of Logan. US 89 deserves every bit of its status as a National Scenic Byway. This winding highway makes a dramatic cut through a gorgeous portion of Uinta-Wasatch-Cache National Forest, demanding the full attention of every driver as it climbs and clings to towering canyon walls and carves through the cliffs high above the Logan River below.

Lodge Campground is a refuge from all this ruggedness—a safe haven found on a small detour up the right fork of the Logan River. This is not to say that Lodge isn't spectacular; indeed, it is in its own way. While most of its siblings host larger camping crowds (Guinavah-Malibu, for instance, has 40 individual sites), the real charm of Lodge lies in the fact that it has just 10 sites.

Each site has just what you need—not too much, not too little: a picnic table, a fire ring, a parking spot, and a plot to plop your tent on. Water spigots are dispersed throughout camp, but note that some may be turned off depending on the time of year.

The Logan Canyon Scenic Byway rewards travelers with spectacular views.

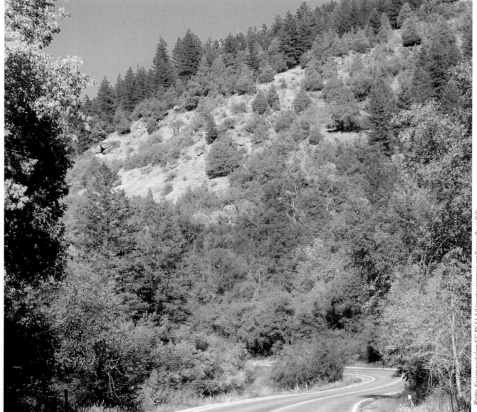

KEY INFORMATION

LOCATION: FR 047, Logan, UT 84321

CONTACT: 435-755-3620, tinyurl.com
/uwcnfcamping

OPERATED BY: American Land & Leisure for
Uinta-Wasatch-Cache National Forest,
Logan Ranger District

OPEN: June–October

SITES: 10

EACH SITE: Picnic table, fire ring

ASSIGNMENT: First-come, first-served;
no reservations

REGISTRATION: On-site self-registration

AMENITIES: Vault toilets, drinking water,
firewood

PARKING: At campsites only

FEES: $17/night, $8/extra vehicle

WHEELCHAIR ACCESS: Not designated

ELEVATION: 5,457'

RESTRICTIONS:

PETS: On leash only

FIRES: In fire rings only

ALCOHOL: Permitted

VEHICLES: Up to 34 feet

OTHER: 7-day stay limit; maximum
8 people/site

The campground is laid out in a typical loop: sites 1–4 on the stem, 5–10 on the bend. Site 7 may have a slight edge over the others when it comes to privacy and spaciousness, but that's nitpicking, really: there's not a bad site in the bunch.

In contrast to the bigger campgrounds on the main highway, you'll find abundant peace and quiet at Lodge. Not only are you off the main road, but Lodge also remains somewhat undiscovered, or at least unfavored. The only exception to peace and quiet would be traffic coming to and from Camp LoMia, a privately owned youth camp just a few hundred yards away. You may catch a drop-off or pick-up day and have plenty of company, but don't fret: the commotion is only temporary, and peace and quiet return in short order.

Shade abounds in and around the campground—a good thing, because at just shy of 5,500 feet, Lodge doesn't cool down as quickly as camps farther up the canyon. On the bright side, the warmer weather at this elevation means that Lodge can open earlier and close later than many other Logan-area camping spots.

As you drive up Logan Canyon, you may think to yourself that the Logan River looks like a great place to fling a fly. You'd be absolutely right! From the third dam on the river up to the Idaho state line, the Logan River is designated as a Blue Ribbon Fishery. This distinction comes with a price, however, as crowds are heavy and special restrictions apply. Don't let that deter you, though; there's plenty of river for everyone, and even kids can get in on the action a little lower at one of the impoundments closer to Logan City.

The Right Fork of the Logan River, which runs near the campground, is a fun place to fish in its own right. Again, it's not as big or brassy as the Logan proper, but it is decently fishable.

If you take US 89 for 30 more miles to the end of the Logan Canyon Scenic Byway, you'll find yourself at Bear Lake. A few camping spots are scattered near the lake, but this is a great place to just spend the day even if you're based at Lodge. Water levels at Bear Lake fluctuate considerably depending on the time of year and how wet previous winters have been, but this is usually a pretty reliable place to hook into some Bear Lake cutthroat trout. This strain of Bonneville cutthroat evolved in Bear Lake and now prospers in its alkaline waters.

Bear Lake is also famous for its raspberries, and in Garden City you'll find plenty of places to partake of them. If they're in season, bring some home for the neighbors and you'll be a hero for years. Don't miss the opportunity to try a homemade raspberry shake, either—it's so tasty, most people have a hard time eating one slowly enough to avoid a brain freeze. Be strong. Take your time. Savor the flavor; save a few brain cells. You may like it so much that you'll have to get one on the way into town and another on the way out.

Logan residents who haven't yet discovered Lodge Campground will value its accessibility. Outsiders will welcome the straightforward layout and simple setup. Either way, the baby of the Logan Canyon campground family does the region proud.

Lodge Campground

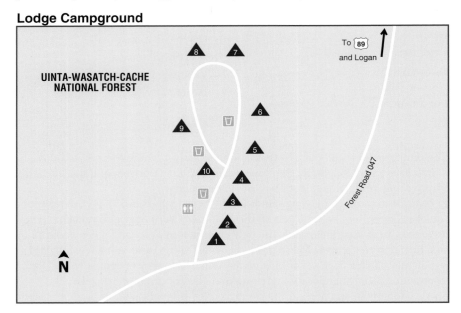

GETTING THERE

From the intersection of North Main Street and UT 89 (East 400 North) in Logan, go 11 miles east up Logan Canyon on US 89. Then, just after the road crosses the Logan River, turn right onto Forest Road 081, following the signs for Camp LoMia. Continue 1.3 miles on FR 081, and then turn right onto FR 047; Lodge Campground is immediately ahead on your right, just after you cross the Right Fork of the Logan River and just before Camp LoMia on your left.

GPS COORDINATES: N41° 46.646' W111° 37.217'

16

Maple Canyon Campground

Beauty: ★★★★ / Privacy: ★★★★ / Quiet: ★★★★ / Spaciousness: ★★★★ / Security: ★★★★★ /
Cleanliness: ★★★★

Maple Canyon makes rock climbers feel like kids in a candy store.

The pockmarked cobble walls of Maple Canyon plunge down and meet the ground as if they had thrown down the gauntlet and challenged you to climb them. Rock climbers from all over the state—and even the country—are answering that challenge and confirming that this is one of the best places in the world to climb cobblestone. By day they conquer cliffs, but by night they sleep at Maple Canyon Campground.

There are 16 sites in a string, just inside the Manti–La Sal National Forest boundary west of the farming town of Moroni. Only one small sign indicates the campground's presence, a brown blur on UT 132 near Fountain Green.

The first of these sites in Maple Canyon is designed to hold groups of up to 40 people. Sites 2–4 are individual sites strung along a spur off the main campground road, are walk-in only, and are probably the best sites in camp privacy-wise. Because of the high canyon walls, sunshine is at a premium. Sites 5–9 give you the most minutes of sunshine each day, which is probably worth considering if you stay here during spring or fall. Sites 10–16 sit at the top of the campground, far away from the nine below them. Site 12 is also walk-in only.

All of the sites at Maple Canyon can be reserved. If the group site isn't being occupied, it's offered on a first-come, first-served basis at $40 per night. The other sites are also up for

Rock climbers in Maple Canyon

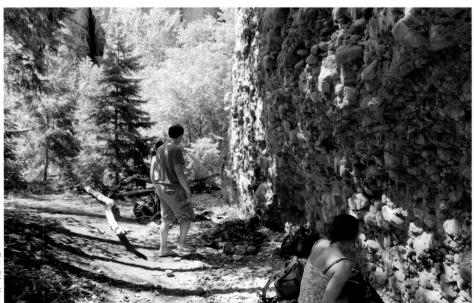

Photo: Richard Luong

KEY INFORMATION

LOCATION: FR 0066, Moroni, UT 84646

CONTACTS: 435-283-4151, tinyurl.com
/mantilasalcamping; reservations: 877-444-
6777, recreation.gov

OPERATED BY: Manti–La Sal National Forest,
Sanpete Ranger District

OPEN: May–October

SITES: 15 (including 4 walk-ins), plus
1 group site

EACH SITE: Picnic table, fire ring,
barbecue stand

ASSIGNMENT: First-come, first-served and
by reservation

REGISTRATION: On-site self-registration
or online

AMENITIES: Vault toilets

PARKING: At campsites only

FEES: $8/night (single), $40/night (group)

WHEELCHAIR ACCESS: Not designated

ELEVATION: 6,803'

RESTRICTIONS:

PETS: On leash only

FIRES: In fire rings only

ALCOHOL: Permitted

VEHICLES: Up to 35 feet

OTHER: 14-day stay limit; maximum
6 or 8 people/site (single) or 40 people/
site (group)

grabs when they're not already spoken for, but it only takes a moment to make a reservation, so why not do it?

The restrooms are vault toilets, but they're sturdy and neat. Water isn't available at camp, but there's a small trickle of a stream that runs adjacent to the road where you can pump and purify. Bring plenty of your own water in case the stream is dry.

What's not cobbled cliff walls or sandy light brown earth is probably a maple tree. A few evergreens dot the landscape here and there, but most of the green comes from maple trees of every size. For being so close to the Sanpete Valley floor, the canyon is much greener than you'd expect.

Maple Canyon makes rock climbers feel like kids in a candy store. The sheer number and variety of routes available are enough to earn this canyon a reputation as one of the world's best places to climb. An entire book has been written about just this canyon, detailing the different areas to climb, but any gear shop around should be able to point the uninitiated in the right direction.

Difficulty levels range from beginner to hardcore routes for the most insane climbers. Among the most climbed are Engagement Alcove and the Schoolroom, although there are countless climbs known by many names in the area.

Ice climbing is also quite popular in Maple Canyon, but the conditions aren't always favorable. Your best bet would be to hop online and find other climbers in the area who may have a recent report. The campground closes in the wintertime, but ice climbers spend the precious daylight hours tied to the sheer ice walls that form.

Rock climbing isn't the only game in town. Take one of the trails that connect to the side canyons—one to the north and one to the south. They're only short trails that take off right near the campground, but they will give you a hint of the real personality of the canyons of the San Pitch Mountains.

The San Pitch range marks the border between Sanpete and Juab Counties. Although these mountains aren't especially tall, they rise above the Sanpete Valley and offer convenient camping to residents on both sides. Trails and rough roads snake throughout the range. In fact, it's possible to drive from Wales to Levan on Forest Road 101. Find the road by going back out to Westside Road and going south 4 miles to Wales, then turning right. Wales Canyon will lift you up over the ridge of the San Pitch Range, then the road will funnel you back down along Chicken Creek.

I'm not much of a rock climber myself, but I still find Maple Canyon fascinating. Every texture, every color, and every little side canyon is so different, yet they somehow blend together to make it work.

Maple Canyon Campground

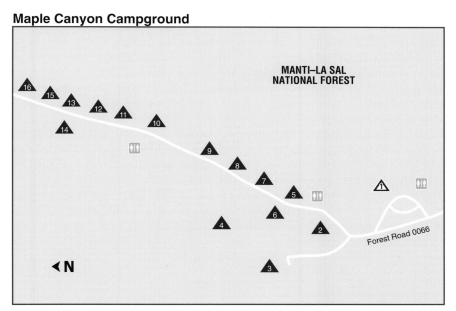

GETTING THERE

From the intersection of South 400 East (UT 132) and East Main Street (UT 116) in the town of Moroni, head west 0.7 mile on Main Street; then bear left at the fork onto West 17200 North. In 2.6 miles, turn right (north) onto West Side Road. Go 1.3 miles and turn left onto Freedom Road; in another 0.5 mile, turn right onto Maple Canyon Road (FR 0066) and drive north another 3 miles to the campground.

GPS COORDINATES: N39° 33.361' W111° 41.184'

17

Maple Grove Campground

Beauty: ★★★★ / Privacy: ★★★★ / Quiet: ★★★★ / Spaciousness: ★★★★ / Security: ★★★★ /
Cleanliness: ★★★★★

Maple Grove is where the locals camp.

All great campgrounds can be found in the same place: the last place you'd look for them. This little nugget of wisdom will lead you to some of the most surprising and wonderful campgrounds in *any* state, and it certainly holds true in Utah. Case in point: Maple Grove.

This calm and flourishing sanctuary is located on the foothills of the Pahvant Range between Scipio and Aurora. Don't feel bad if you're not sure where any of those places are, because not many people do. Fish Lake seems to get all the publicity in Fishlake National Forest (gee, I wonder why?), meaning the Pahvant Range, Tushar Mountains, and Sevier Plateau stay blissfully unadvertised. There are a handful of campgrounds in these parts of Fishlake just like Maple Grove—relatively unknown and unspoiled.

Maple Grove has two parts: first, the main loop with individual sites 1–14, and second, three piggybacking loops with group sites A–C. The main loop is separated from the group sites by lovely little Ivie (sometimes spelled Ivy) Creek, which begins between sites 14 and 20 as it bubbles up from the ground and gurgles its way down the hillside.

Each site is well spaced, with good access to one of three water spigots on the loop, but be prepared to do a little extra walking every time you need to use the potty if you stay along the back of the loop (sites 5–11 or thereabouts). Long-distance potty trot or not, numbers 7 and 9 are appropriated a bit more space and privacy than their neighbors. The incontinent can take site 1—also private and very near the restroom.

Cascades on Ivie Creek

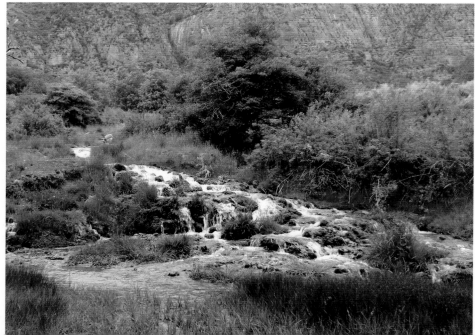

KEY INFORMATION

LOCATION: Along Ivie Creek about 4 miles west of US 50, Fillmore, UT 84631

CONTACTS: 435-743-5721, tinyurl.com/fishlakenfcamping; reservations: 877-444-6777, recreation.gov, or reserveamerica.com

OPERATED BY: Fishlake National Forest, Fillmore Ranger District

OPEN: May–October

SITES: 20, plus 3 group sites

EACH SITE: Picnic table, fire ring, barbecue stand

ASSIGNMENT: First-come, first-served; group sites by reservation

REGISTRATION: On-site self-registration or online (group sites)

AMENITIES: Vault toilets, drinking water

PARKING: At campsites only

FEES: $15/night (single), $50/night (group site B), $70/night (group site A), $90/night (group site C), $7.50 extra vehicle

WHEELCHAIR ACCESS: Some individual sites; all group sites and restrooms

ELEVATION: 6,486'

RESTRICTIONS:

PETS: On leash only

FIRES: In fire rings only

ALCOHOL: Permitted

VEHICLES: Up to 40 feet

OTHER: 14-day stay limit; maximum 8 people/site (single), 56 people/site (group site B), 96 people/site (group site A), or 100 people/site (group site C), no firewood gathering; off-road vehicles prohibited

I asked the campground host there to describe the typical Maple Grove guest. Without hesitation, he replied, "Locals. This is where the locals camp."

To his point, this is one of those campgrounds that aren't really stopping points on the way *to* anywhere or hot destinations in themselves. When the locals want to get away for some peace and quiet, this is where they come. And why not? The canopy created by the maples creates a protective shell against the outside world. And along this stretch of US 50, there's not a lot of outside world knocking at the door.

The locals take good care of Maple Grove. The tables show few signs of use, and the trees and bushes surrounding the campsite are in good shape. The gravel road is likewise in great condition and makes this campground accessible to just about anyone—that does include RVs, although I wouldn't worry too much about noise. Respect extends beyond the maintenance of the grounds to the folks who camp on them.

Ivie Creek is planted a couple of times each year with rainbow and brown trout catchables, mostly for kids during the summer. They get pretty wily pretty quick (the trout, that is), so don't think you're going to have any easy hookups with unwitting hatchery fish. Just be patient—that's the happy fisherman's motto.

Ivie Creek creates a spectacular waterfall about a quarter mile back down Maple Grove Road. You'd kick yourself for missing it—pull off toward the river about the time you see an open area with tire tracks on the north side of the road. Just beyond the trees and top lip of the river embankment, a small trail leads down to the river below the gorgeous cascade. You're pushing the boundaries of U.S. Forest Service property here, so watch for posted NO TRESPASSING signs.

Bring your camera to capture this magnificent display of tumbling water. Rather than crashing down in a single forceful plunge, the watery fingers of the falls crawl between rocks and over lush green grasses before tumbling down to small pools, collecting and slowly moving back down to the valley floor. It's mesmerizing.

Many campers come to Maple Grove to access the Paiute ATV Trail, which traverses a huge chunk of Fishlake National Forest. Off-road vehicles are prohibited in the campground proper, though, so you won't have to contend with buzzing motors when you're trying to sleep in. (If you want to ride, a number of outfitters in the area rent ATVs.)

Trails leave from camp and eventually meet back up with Forest Road 096. You can take the road north to scale Coffee Peak or south to try Jacks Peak. Both are just over 10,000 feet in elevation and will let you peek over the Pahvant Range to see the Sevier Desert to the west. Frankly, you could wander around exploring side canyons for days, crisscrossing the Paiute trail the whole way through.

Maple Grove Campground

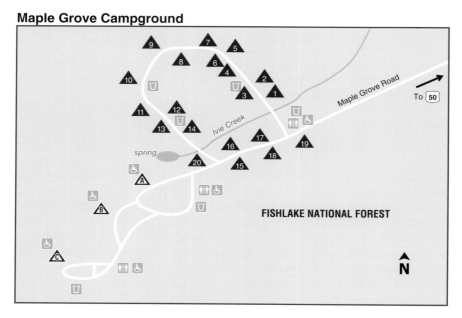

GETTING THERE

From I-15, take Exit 188 in Scipio, about 122 miles south of Salt Lake City. About 0.5 mile off the exit ramp, turn right (south) onto US 50 (North Main Street). Drive 15.5 miles southeast on US 50; then turn right (west) onto Maple Grove Road—look for the cattle gate and brown campground sign. In 1.8 miles, turn left onto North 9200 East and follow the road 2.2 miles south and west to the campground, on your right at the end of the road.

GPS COORDINATES: N39° 1.109' W112° 5.341'

18

⚠ Mill Hollow Campground

Beauty: ★★★★★ / Privacy: ★★★ / Quiet: ★★★★ / Spaciousness: ★★★★ / Security: ★★★★ /
Cleanliness: ★★★★

A combination of great attributes makes this little spot a must-try for Utah tenters.

There are no superlatives at Mill Hollow—it's not the highest, biggest, or most beautiful campground you'll find. But that doesn't mean it's mediocre. In fact, it's the combination of great attributes that makes this little spot a must-see for Utah tenters.

Climbing the dirt road off UT 35 is a lesson in suspense. The road whips back and forth over graded (but washboard) dirt and never lets you see Mill Hollow Reservoir until you're within spitting distance. Then you take an easy left over the dam and find yourself in this hearty forest campground, on the shores of the light-blue reservoir.

There are two simple loops: the elongated Loop A with sites 1–13, and the rounder, shorter Loop B with sites 14–28. Decidedly more spread out, Loop A has hiking access to the waterfront from a few of its sites. Specifically, sites 1–5 will get you closest, and site 5 is the most exclusive of the bunch.

Some sites accommodate RVs, but there are plenty that don't have a driveway and are better suited for tenters. The dense forest setting will help screen you from your neighbors. If you're concerned about getting a site that suits your tenting needs, 11 sites are currently designated as tent-only: 5, 7, 9, 10, 13, 14, 18–20, 23, and 24.

The campground's namesake reservoir

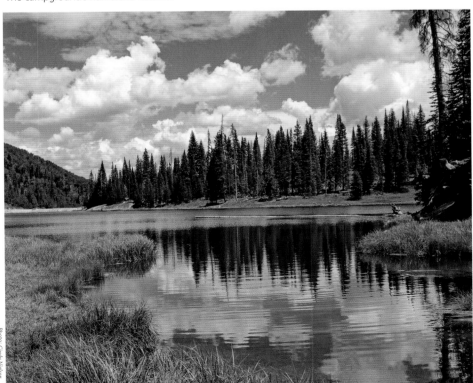

KEY INFORMATION

LOCATION: South of FR 054, Heber City, UT 84032

CONTACTS: 435-654-0470, tinyurl.com /uwcnfcamping; reservations: 877-444-6777, recreation.gov

OPERATED BY: Uinta-Wasatch-Cache National Forest, Heber-Kamas Ranger District

OPEN: July–October

SITES: 28

EACH SITE: Picnic table, fire ring, grill

ASSIGNMENT: First-come, first-served and by reservation

REGISTRATION: On-site self-registration or online

AMENITIES: Vault toilets, drinking water

PARKING: At campsites only

FEE: $20/night

WHEELCHAIR ACCESS: Restrooms only

ELEVATION: 8,887'

RESTRICTIONS:

PETS: Leashed

FIRES: In fire rings only

ALCOHOL: Permitted

VEHICLES: Up to 50 feet

OTHER: 7-day stay limit; maximum 8 people, 1 vehicle/site; off-road vehicles prohibited

In the farming- and ranching-heavy West, where "whiskey is for drinking and water is for fighting," Mill Hollow Reservoir is something of an odd duck. Created in 1962, it's maintained by the Department of Wildlife Resources and Uinta-Wasatch-Cache National Forest for recreational use. Where many other reservoirs capture water from early-spring runoff and release it slowly over the course of the summer for irrigation, water is never released from Mill Hollow for agriculture.

As a result, this is a tremendously popular family fishery. Crowds are heavy, but the hatchery truck makes frequent stops to deposit catchable-sized rainbow, brook, and tiger trout. From the end of June through August, the lake is planted about once a week with one or more of those species, which average about 10 inches at planting time. While the reservoir has winter-killed in the past, most years it does not, and any holdovers will start reaching the 14- and 15-inch-plus range. That's no state record, but when little Tommy cranks in a 15-inch rainbow, he'll think it's the biggest fish that's ever flapped a gill.

Mill Hollow is also well suited to canoes and rafts. There is a crude boat launch, although no motors are allowed. If you just can't seem to find the fish from shore, or if the kids can't cast beyond the algae "gunk" that seems to form each season, bring your trusty vessel and paddle around to find an open space.

Explore the Mill Hollow Trail, which leaves from the campground near site 16, to get better views of the surrounding canyon. After a few hundred yards, the trail splits and lets you decide how tough you're feeling. Both directions will complete the loop, but the one on the left will take you through lodgepole pine and provides a more gradual ascent, while the fork to the right is much steeper and shorter. After you summit near a stand of aspens, the trail descends over steep terrain back down toward the campground, passing a small marshy area and joining a double-track road. While the trail is open to mountain bikes, they're not recommended because of the rough terrain.

If you continue on Forest Road 054, keep straight until it becomes FR 094 and meets FR 050. You'll hook around on FR 050 and drop into the very beginnings of the west fork of the

Duchesne River. Although it begins as just a trickle, you can follow the river as it picks up momentum from other small tributaries and local springs. By the time you've gone a couple of miles, it's turned into a bona fide waterway, teeming with little trout.

As close as Mill Hollow is to the Wasatch Front and all it has to offer, it's a surprise that the campground isn't filled to capacity every night. Take advantage of this resource built for the very purpose of your recreation. You'll be glad you did.

Mill Hollow Campground

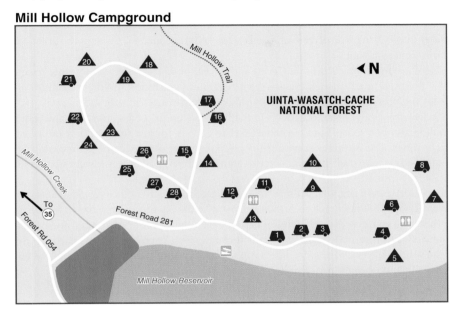

GETTING THERE

From the intersection of UT 35 and Bench Creek Road in the town of Woodland, go 11 miles southeast on UT 35 and turn right onto FR 054. Drive south 2.8 miles; then turn left into the campground on FR 281.

GPS COORDINATES: N40° 29.424' W111° 6.223'

19

Monte Cristo Campground

Beauty: ★★★★ / Privacy: ★★★★ / Quiet: ★★★ / Spaciousness: ★★★★ / Security: ★★★ / Cleanliness: ★★★★★

One of this campground's best features is the symphony of scents in the air at any given time.

Few campgrounds can rival Monte Cristo for that woodsy feeling. Planted high in the Monte Cristo Mountain Range, the campground operates for just a few short months from mid-summer into fall, but year after year families keep coming back for the superb surroundings and fresh mountain air.

There are five loops at Monte Cristo and a total of 47 campsites. Only sites 26 and 27 can be reserved in advance; these are the group sites, which each hold a maximum of 100 people. The remaining sites are available only on a first-come, first-served basis.

Ordinarily, a campground with 45 individual sites up for grabs gives you a decent shot at finding an open space. Because Monte Cristo is open for just three to four months each year, however, the camping season gets condensed and sites become scarce on a Friday afternoon. This is a wildly popular place to camp, and for good reason, so get up there early to stake out your site.

Loop A or B will suit you just fine. Loop C is a good second choice. You'll probably want to avoid Loops D and E if possible; they're closest to the big group sites and sit a little closer together than you may prefer. Each site has its own picnic table and fire ring, and only a few of the sites accommodate big RVs in pull-through sites. There's no river nearby to drown out the sounds of your neighbors, but if you're choosy about your campsite, you'll be able to employ the "out of sight, out of mind" principle.

Woodsy Monte Cristo fills up fast, so stake out your site well ahead of time.

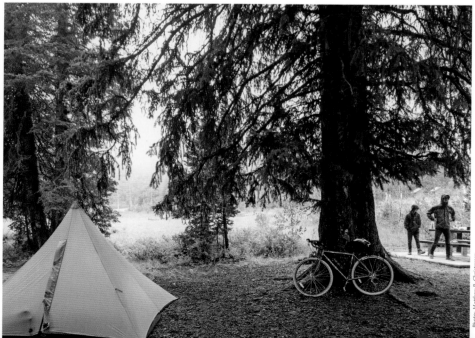

Photo: Matthew B. Christensen

KEY INFORMATION

LOCATION: FR 20064 just off UT 39, Ogden, UT 84401

CONTACTS: 801-625-5306, tinyurl.com/uwcnfcamping; reservations: 877-444-6777, recreation.gov

OPERATED BY: Uinta-Wasatch-Cache National Forest, Ogden Ranger District

OPEN: July–October

SITES: 45, plus 2 group sites

EACH SITE: Picnic table, fire ring

ASSIGNMENT: First-come, first-served; group sites by reservation

REGISTRATION: On-site self-registration or online (group sites)

AMENITIES: Vault toilets, drinking water, garbage service

PARKING: At campsites only

FEES: $20/night (single), $180/night (group), $8/additional vehicle, $6 walk-in fee

WHEELCHAIR ACCESS: Not designated

ELEVATION: 8,947'

RESTRICTIONS:

PETS: On leash only

FIRES: In fire rings only

ALCOHOL: Permitted

VEHICLES: Up to 45 feet

OTHER: 7-day stay limit; maximum 8 people/site (single) or 100 people/site (group)

One big reason for Monte Cristo's popularity is its location—not just where it sits in the state, but where it sits on the mountain. Ogden and Weber County residents favor this place for its proximity to home. It's only an hour or so from Ogden, but in terms of atmosphere, it's a world away.

Other fine campgrounds can be found along the way, especially between Pineview Reservoir and the junction with Causey Road. In fact, if UT 39 is still closed from winter, there's a chance that one of these lower campgrounds will be open. Campers love that when UT 39 finally does open, there's a sheltered campground at 9,000 feet, right off the highway, shaded by beautiful aspens and enormous evergreens.

One of the best things about Monte Cristo is the symphony of scents in the air at any given time. Whether it's after a rainstorm (somewhat common in these parts) or at dinnertime when families are cooking supper, the air here is always delicious. With the convenience of drinking water and garbage service, you can pack along the ingredients to the most elaborate camping fare and help contribute to the blend of splendid outdoor smells. Intoxicating!

Although there's no shortage of things to do, most people who stay at Monte Cristo really *stay* at Monte Cristo. The only deterrent you might have to lounging around your campsite would be the flies and mosquitoes. Some years are worse than others, but that just means the difference between bringing one or two cans of bug juice. You've been warned.

If you do have the willpower to break out of your Monte Cristo "aroma coma," drive to Birch Creek, about 12 miles away on UT 39 toward Woodruff. Two small reservoirs sitting about a mile off the highway are great places to dunk a worm. There's also a small campground with four walk-in sites operated by the Bureau of Land Management if you just can't deal with the crowds at Monte Cristo.

Continue 2 more miles down UT 39 and turn off to Woodruff Creek Reservoir for similar recreational opportunities, minus the campground. This reservoir's water levels fluctuate greatly as the summer progresses, so expect muddy shores as fall approaches.

The Monte Cristo Range is full of back roads, byways, and little trails. As you drive along UT 39, duck into one of these turnoffs (once you've passed the private-property segment) to see where it takes you. I took a trail just southwest of camp and found a cleared meadow that gave me incomparable views. I ended up snapping a remarkable photograph of the sunset, just as it dipped behind the mountains in the distance.

In the wintertime, this area is a snowmobiling mecca. Ant Flat and Forest Road 054 (just below the gate that closes UT 39 when snow gets too deep) are buzzing with action. Monte Cristo Campground is closed in winter, but that shouldn't stop you from heading up by sled or snowshoe and smelling that crisp winter mountain air.

Monte Cristo Campground

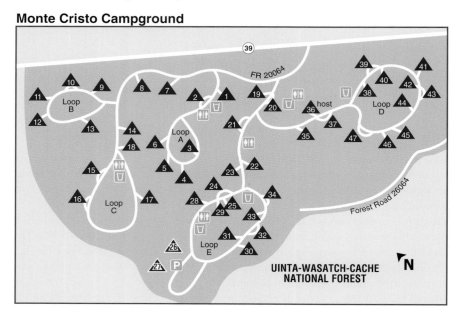

GETTING THERE

From the intersection of UT 16 and UT 39 in Woodruff, go 20.2 miles southwest on UT 39 (Ogden River Scenic Byway) to the campground, on your left.

GPS COORDINATES: N41° 27.822' W111° 29.862'

20

Pioneer Campground

Beauty: ★★★★ / Privacy: ★★★★ / Quiet: ★★★★ / Spaciousness: ★★★ / Security: ★★★ / Cleanliness: ★★★★

On the banks of the Blacksmith Fork, this is the picture-perfect campground to capitalize on the recreation offered by the river.

The Blacksmith Fork River isn't that different from other rivers, yet it has a personality all its own, its clear waters rolling softly and gently down an out-of-the-way canyon. Pioneer Campground, on the banks of the Blacksmith Fork, is the picture-perfect campground to capitalize on the recreational opportunities offered by the river.

This campground has two sections, with most sites located on the main loop away from the road. After site 2, a quirky little spur takes off to the right and leads to sites 3, 4, and 5. The best of this group is site 3, which backs up into nothing but vegetation; sites 4 and 5 share boundaries with campsites along the main road. On the other fork of the road, between sites 1 and 2, are sites 16–18. They're far removed from the main camping area, so if you're trying to get three sites together for a larger group, this setup is perfect. If it's just you, choose site 17 for its distance from the others and its position right on the river.

Secluded Blacksmith Fork Canyon provides a striking setting for this campground.

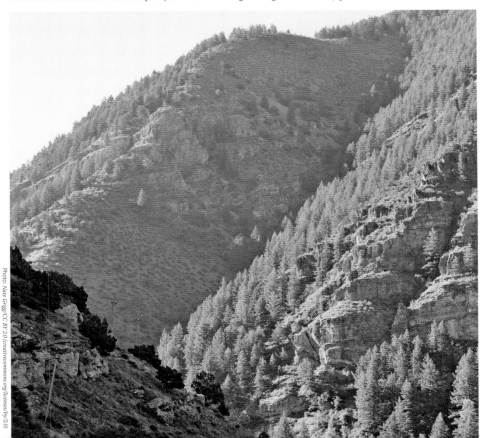

KEY INFORMATION

LOCATION: FR 155 just south of UT 101, Hyrum, UT 84319

CONTACT: 435-755-3620, tinyurl.com/uwcnf camping

OPERATED BY: American Land & Leisure for Uinta-Wasatch-Cache National Forest, Logan Ranger District

OPEN: May–September

SITES: 18

EACH SITE: Picnic table, fire ring

ASSIGNMENT: First-come, first-served; no reservations

REGISTRATION: On-site self-registration

AMENITIES: Vault toilets, drinking water, garbage service

PARKING: At campsites only

FEES: $17/night, $8/extra vehicle

WHEELCHAIR ACCESS: Not designated

ELEVATION: 5,086'

RESTRICTIONS:

PETS: On leash only

FIRES: In fire rings only

ALCOHOL: Permitted

VEHICLES: Up to 34 feet

OTHER: 7-day stay limit; maximum 8 people/site

The Blacksmith Fork is locally renowned as a trout stream. It is designated as a Blue Ribbon Fishery, a distinction awarded by the US government to rivers and streams with excellent water quality and quantity, accessibility to anglers, optimal environmental conditions for sustaining a healthy fish population, the ability to accommodate fishing crowds without sacrificing the quality of the recreational experience, and the presence of certain fish species. The 16-mile stretch from the first impoundment excels in each of these criteria, and at Pioneer you're right in the thick of things.

The river is known for its large, lumbering turns and gentle riffles. Mostly brown trout swim these waters, so nymphing and streamers seem to be most productive. Bait fishing is allowed, so even the most impatient 6-year-old can have a shot at a brown or even the occasional cutthroat or mountain whitefish. Note that the river passes through some stretches of private land—river access is limited here, but such areas are generally well signed.

In recent years, an overabundance of brown trout has depleted the Blacksmith Fork's population of forage (bait) fish; to help keep the river's ecosystem in balance, anglers are encouraged to harvest browns to thin the herd. Check the current *Utah Fishing Guidebook* (available as a free download at wildlife.utah.gov/utah-fishing-guidebook.html) or wildlife .utah.gov/hotspots for the latest information—biologists are always monitoring the water, and conditions can change quickly.

If the main river is too crowded, try a detour up the Left Hand Fork; Forest Road 055 will take you to areas with good public access. This is also a good backup plan if Pioneer is full—there are a couple of places to camp along the road.

Hikers will be in hog heaven (pun intended) up FR 055. Just east of Spring Campground is the trailhead access for a hike to four springs: Hog Hole, Pig Hole, Boar Hole, and Sow Hole. This easy loop is bound to delight everyone down to the most dedicated vegetarian.

Just 7 miles east of camp is Hardware Ranch. While the name may conjure images of wild screwdrivers and free-range nuts and bolts, the main creatures you'll find here are elk. The state of Utah purchased the ranch in 1945 from the Box Elder Hardware Company and established it as a place to study and manage local elk herds, especially in winter months.

Elk have historically come down Blacksmith Fork Canyon into the Cache Valley to feed during the winter, but by the early 20th century, homes and farms were starting to squeeze them out. Hardware Ranch was set up as a winter range for the elk, and each year the state grows tons of grass hay for the foraging herds.

If you're staying at Pioneer, that probably means it's still relatively warm outside and the 500–600 elk that frequent the ranch haven't yet taken up residence. Still, you can drop in at the visitor center to learn more about elk and other wildlife near the ranch through interactive displays and staff programs. If you plan to visit during the winter, mark your calendar for the annual Hardware Ranch Elk Festival, which offers sleigh rides each winter through the elk feeding grounds. Check wildlife.utah.gov/hardwareranch for details.

Pioneer Campground

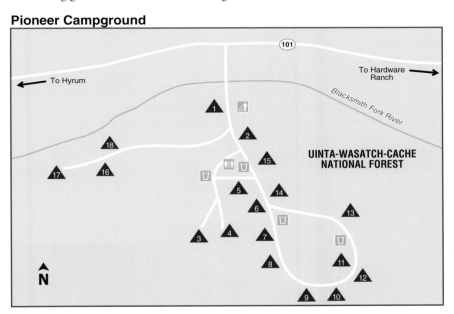

GETTING THERE

From the intersection of UT 165 (800 East) and UT 101 (Blacksmith Fork Canyon Road) in Hyrum, drive 8 miles east on UT 101 and, at the brown sign on your left, turn right to reach the campground.

GPS COORDINATES: N41° 37.733' W111° 41.560'

21

Ponderosa Campground

Beauty: ★★★★ / Privacy: ★★★ / Quiet: ★★★★ / Spaciousness: ★★★ / Security: ★★★★ / Cleanliness: ★★★

With towering peaks, cool crystalline creeks, and thick swaths of forest, this just might be your promised land.

In the Old Testament, Moses goes up to Mount Nebo after wandering in the wilderness, and he sees the Promised Land, but he is told he'll never get to go there. If you visit Utah's Mount Nebo Wilderness, your experience may be quite different: you may think you've already made it. With towering peaks, cool crystalline creeks, and thick swatches of forest, this might just be *your* promised land.

Planted just outside the official Mount Nebo Wilderness boundary is Ponderosa Campground with its 23 campsites. I hope I look as good at 85 as Ponderosa does, although it's obvious this campground has had some work done. The picnic tables and fire rings are now cast in cement, but the traditional square of cement has been forgone in favor of more organic, rounded shapes that soften the look and complement the curves of Mother Nature. A small sign pays homage to the "visionary men" who planted ponderosa pines here in 1914, almost 20 years before an official campground was constructed in 1933.

Ponderosa pines give this campground not only its name but also its personality. Their tall, slender trunks shoot up out of an otherwise scrubby landscape. At their feet, the ground is littered with pine needles and the occasional grassy patch, but it remains remarkably flat

The Nebo Loop is the state's premier leaf-peeping route in the fall.

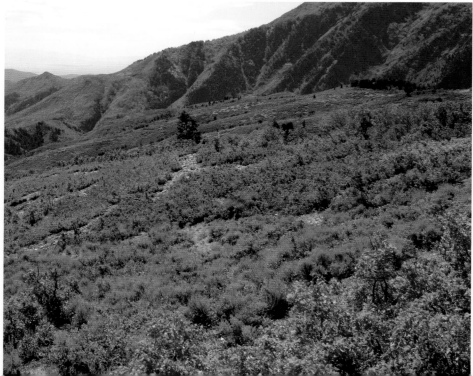

Photo: GylasDigiPhoto/Shutterstock

KEY INFORMATION

LOCATION: FR 048, Nephi, UT 84648

CONTACTS: 801-798-3571, tinyurl.com /uwcnfcamping; reservations: 877-444-6777, recreation.gov

OPERATED BY: American Land & Leisure for Uinta-Wasatch-Cache National Forest, Spanish Fork Ranger District

OPEN: May–October

SITES: 23

EACH SITE: Picnic table, fire ring

ASSIGNMENT: First-come, first-served and by reservation

REGISTRATION: On-site self-registration or online

AMENITIES: Vault toilets, drinking water

PARKING: At campsites only

FEES: $18/night, $8/extra vehicle; $8 day-use fee

WHEELCHAIR ACCESS: Not designated

ELEVATION: 6,203'

RESTRICTIONS:

PETS: On leash only

FIRES: In fire rings only

ALCOHOL: Permitted

VEHICLES: Up to 110 feet

OTHER: 16-day stay limit; maximum 8 people/site; gates close at 10 p.m.; off-road vehicles and horses prohibited

and even, so you won't have to worry about setting up your tent on a slope and waking up nose to nose with your tent buddy. Beyond the campground in both directions, the plant life is a little more typical of what you might find at this elevation: thick brush, oak, and the occasional lonely evergreen.

Ponderosa pines are great for shade, but they don't do a great job at providing privacy. They're typically branchless from at least eye level down, so there's no solid shield between you and your neighbors. Fortunately, these individual sites aren't stacked right on top of each other. Pick the right site, position your tent just so, and you'll find enough privacy to get by.

Two-thirds of the sites here can be reserved ahead of time, while sites 1, 5, 7, 8, 10, 17, and 21 are offered on a first-come, first-served basis. Of the reservables, site 6 offers the most space and backs up into Salt Creek to drown out any unwanted noise. If you're rolling the dice and plan on just showing up to look for a site, try site 8 for all the same reasons as site 6. Both happen to be on the right loop of the campground, but there's nothing wrong with exploring the left loop, which holds sites 14–23.

Not too many people spend the night in one of the Nebo Loop area campgrounds, but plenty of Utahns drive the area during the day, especially in the fall. The Nebo Loop National Scenic Byway (Forest Road 015), or the Nebo Loop for short, is arguably Utah's most famous route for viewing fall foliage. The 32-mile stretch of paved road lifts drivers to more than 9,000 feet in elevation and passes giant groves of maple, oak, and aspen that are woven together in the heart of this section of Uinta-Wasatch-Cache National Forest. Each fall they ignite into a spectacular show of pure reds, brilliant yellows, creamy oranges, and every shade and mixture in between. The Nebo Loop also shows off the dark-blue waters of the Payson Lakes (an incredible but crowded camping area), Devil's Kitchen (think a baby Bryce Canyon), and breathtaking views of the valley below. If you take the drive, set aside the entire day. You'll want to stop often for photo ops.

Don't shy away from Ponderosa for fear of long lines of loud cars. The beauty of this campground is that it's located on a small spur of FR 048 off the main Nebo Loop. The most traffic you'll see is the more serious outdoors crowd headed for the hiking near the campground.

Just a mile farther up the road is the Andrews Ridge Trailhead. Catch Trail 117 (Nebo Bench) for a rigorous and demanding trek to the top of Nebo Peak. Considering that the trailhead sits at around 6,500 feet and the peak about a hundred feet shy of 12,000, you're in for quite a hike. Signage pins the one-way ascent at 8 miles, although you'll catch Trail 116 (Nebo Peak) for the last mile and a half. Note that Nebo Peak is different from Mount Nebo: the two sit about a mile away from each other, but there's no official trail to connect them. This is steep and treacherous territory, so use caution along the trail.

If all this seems a little too much, there are plenty of other trails in and around the Mount Nebo Wilderness, including easier routes to the peak. Check the Uinta-Wasatch-Cache National Forest website for excellent route descriptions; go to www.fs.usda.gov/uwcnf and click "Recreation"; then click "Hiking" to access separate lists of overnight and day hikes in each ranger district.

Ponderosa Campground

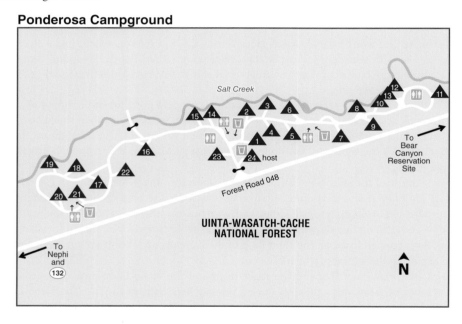

GETTING THERE

From the intersection of Main Street and UT 132 (East 100 North) in Nephi, drive 6 miles east on UT 132 to Nebo Loop Road (FR 015), and bear left at the fork. Go 3.5 miles and bear left another fork onto FR 048; then continue about 0.5 mile to the campground, on your left.

GPS COORDINATES: N39° 46.094' W111° 42.848'

22

Redman Campground

Beauty: ★★★★★ / Privacy: ★★★★ / Quiet: ★★★ / Spaciousness: ★★★★★ / Security: ★★★ /
Cleanliness: ★★★★

You could spend a week at Redman and do something different every day.

The drive to Redman Campground is certainly striking: sheer rock faces full of daring technical climbers, a frothy mountain creek running along one side of the road and then the other, and more recreational areas—including two popular ski resorts—than you can shake a hiking stick at. All of this on your way to the home base of high-mountain camping near Salt Lake City: Redman Campground.

This expansive campground is divided into two main sections: the upper section, tucked into the channel between the highway and Big Cottonwood Creek, and the lower section, on the other side of the river.

The upper section is where you'll find the camp host and, coincidentally, where you'll find most of the action. It's a popular daytime and evening picnic spot, so cars pop in and

This serene meadow in the Wasatch Mountains lies within easy reach of Salt Lake City.

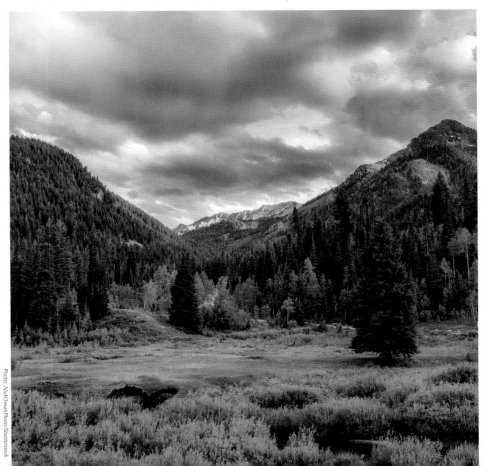

Photo: NickOnanPhoto/Shutterstock

KEY INFORMATION

LOCATION: FR 023 just off UT 190, Solitude, UT 84121

CONTACTS: 801-733-2660, tinyurl.com/uwcnfcamping; reservations: 877-444-6777, recreation.gov

OPERATED BY: American Land & Leisure for Uinta-Wasatch-Cache National Forest, Salt Lake Ranger District

OPEN: Late June–September (depending on weather)

SITES: 36 (including 10 doubles and 2 triples), plus 2 group sites

EACH SITE: Picnic table, fire ring/oven

ASSIGNMENT: First-come, first-served and by reservation

REGISTRATION: On-site self-registration or online

AMENITIES: Vault toilets, drinking water, garbage service

PARKING: At campsites and overflow lot at entrance

FEES: $23/night (single), $46/night (double), $69/night (triple), $110/night (group site 28), $150/night (group site 24), $8/extra vehicle; $8 day-use fee

ELEVATION: 8,350'

WHEELCHAIR ACCESS: Restrooms only

RESTRICTIONS:

PETS: Prohibited

FIRES: In fire rings only

ALCOHOL: Permitted

VEHICLES: Up to 40 feet

OTHER: 7-day stay limit; maximum 8 people/site (single), 16 people/site (double), 24 people/site (triple), 35 people/site (group #28), or 50 people/site (group #24)

out of the campground during most daylight hours. That could be a deal-killer, but Redman's large acreage helps dilute the perceived traffic congestion. Also, the upper-section restrooms have recently been upgraded to modern flush toilets, whereas the lower loop still has a few vault toilets, so the modern facilities of the upper area could be persuasive tools in helping you forget the crowds.

Note: Redman lies within Big Cottonwood Canyon, a protected watershed. Pets are prohibited here.

Several site sizes and capacities are available here. Group site 28 holds 35 people, and group site 24 holds 50. Sites 13, 16, 19, 25, 27, 35, 36, 38, 41, and 44 are all double sites and hold 16 people, for twice the single-site fee. Sites 4-5-6 as well as 7-8-9 are triple sites.

If you want to get away from the buzz, cross the river and pick from campsites 23–49. This lovely bisected loop climbs the hillside and affords some of the more secluded camping in the canyon. If you don't have young children with you, take site 23 and the river will sing you to sleep each night as it passes through the edge of your site. To get as far away from civilization as possible, choose site 38, 43, or 44 on the back side of the loop, where not too many vehicles or people pass.

You can stretch out and relax at Redman, because there's plenty of land to call your own in practically every site. In a canyon dominated by pressure for the development of private property, the USFS deserves kudos for allotting such a large chunk of land to campers. Don't get greedy with the spaciousness, though: limits on the number of people in a given site and the length of vehicles are strictly enforced.

As you enjoy the roominess of your site, look around and take in the scenery. The nearness of Big Cottonwood Creek affords such sights as lush clumps of bright wildflowers and towering pines and aspens. Most campsites have a shady spot somewhere at all hours of the day.

In the mid-1800s, Big Cottonwood Canyon was explored by miners looking for gold, silver, and other precious metals. Today, the real treasure of this backyard canyon is the variety of recreational opportunities it provides. In addition to skiing at Brighton and Solitude Mountain Resorts, the hiking here is top-notch.

Redman sits between the two most popular trailheads in the canyon. Just above the campground, near Brighton Resort, is the boardwalk trail around Silver Lake. This easy stroll around the picturesque pond is accessible to everyone, even providing fishing areas for people with disabilities. For more-serene alpine scenery, leave the boardwalk and climb the mountain trail behind Silver Lake to Twin Lakes, Lake Mary, and Lake Martha on a 5-mile round-trip hike. You can also access Lake Mary from a shorter 1-mile trail that begins from a trailhead behind Wasatch Mountain Lodge.

Another popular hike in Big Cottonwood Canyon begins back down UT 190 at the marked Mill B South Trailhead. Lakes Blanche, Florence, and Lillian will test your grit as you climb about 2,500 feet in less than 4 miles to these icy waters.

Donut Falls, a spectacular waterfall that cascades through a rock "donut," offers one of the most popular hikes in the entire canyon. Kids of all ages can make the short half-mile trek, but watch them closely once you reach the drop into the water below the falls; signs warn of the treacherous and slippery rock. Kudos to Salt Lake City for buying this property from landowners and reopening it to the public once again.

You could spend a week at Redman and do something different every day. Besides offering great hiking and skiing, this area of the Wasatch Mountains is a great place for fishing, mountain biking and climbing, photography, scenic drives, and picnicking. It has even hosted a few kayakers, although Big Cottonwood Creek is inhospitable to anyone but hardcore paddlers.

Redman Campground

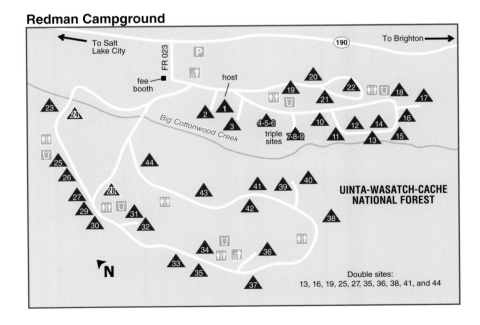

If camp cooking gets old, stop by **Silver Fork Lodge** for breakfast or brunch (11332 Big Cottonwood Canyon Road, Brighton; 801-533-9977, silverforklodge.com). Enjoy your sourdough pancakes while overlooking the pines and aspens, and you'll never want to eat indoors again.

Before you head out to Redman, stop in at the **Public Lands Information Center** of Uinta-Wasatch-Cache National Forest for detailed recreation information (inside REI at 3285 E. 3300 S., Salt Lake City; 801-466-6411). The resources here can help you plan a trip that maximizes all the activities that will be at your fingertips at Redman Campground.

GETTING THERE

From I-15, take Exit 298 in Midvale and head east on 7200 South, which becomes Fort Union Boulevard and then Big Cottonwood Canyon Road/UT 190. After about 20 miles, just past Solitude Mountain Resort, turn right onto Forest Road 023 to reach the campground.

GPS COORDINATES: N40° 36.928' W111° 35.341'

Tanners Flat Campground

Beauty: ★★★★ / Privacy: ★★★★ / Quiet: ★★★ / Spaciousness: ★★★★ / Security: ★★★★ / Cleanliness: ★★★★

Tanners Flat is a welcome break from the hot summers of the city below.

At Tanners Flat Campground in Little Cottonwood Canyon, convenience reigns supreme. Convenient location, convenient campsites, and convenient access to area attractions make this one of the easiest places to stay for your next camping trip.

Just 4 miles up the canyon, Tanners Flat is probably the closest campground to most residents of the southern Salt Lake Valley. Drive to the campground and you'll notice that with each minute, you leave your cares behind and get carried away thinking about the trip ahead. Suburban lawns fade to grassy hillsides, stucco walls give way to sheer rock face, and soon you've gained nearly 3,000 feet in elevation. At 7,250 feet, Tanners Flat is a welcome break from the hot summers of the city below and lends itself to quick getaways designed to beat that heat.

Tanners Flat isn't just convenient for Salt Lake Valley residents. Most camping enthusiasts in Utah County can also make the drive in less than an hour and try something outside of the usual American Fork/Provo Canyon routine.

With camping made so easy, you'd expect Tanners Flat to be packed with people. Well, it is and it isn't. It is literally true that the campground fills up on weekends: a two-day minimum stay is required then, so people come here to settle in, and once it's full, nothing opens until Monday—but at the same time, thick clumps of aspen, oak, and pine form a barrier

This campsite has everything you need for a creekside cookout.

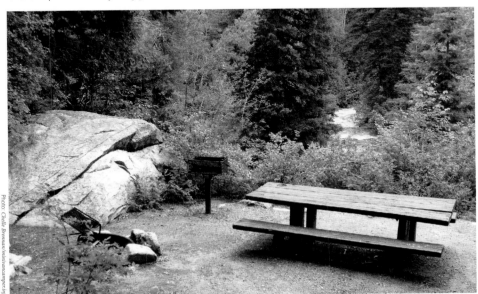

Photo: Chelle Brennan/minivancamper.info

KEY INFORMATION

LOCATION: FR 220 just off UT 210, Sandy, UT 84092

CONTACTS: 801-733-2660, tinyurl.com /uwcnfcamping; reservations: 877-444-6677, recreation.gov

OPERATED BY: American Land & Leisure for Uinta-Wasatch-Cache National Forest, Salt Lake Ranger District

OPEN: Late June–September (depending on weather)

SITES: 35 (including 3 double sites), plus 4 group sites

EACH SITE: Picnic table, fire ring, grill stand

ASSIGNMENT: First-come, first-served and by reservation

REGISTRATION: On-site self-registration and online

AMENITIES: Flush toilets, drinking water, garbage service

PARKING: At campsites and group lots

FEES: $23/night (single), $46/night (double), $90/night (group sites A–C), $150/night (group site D), $8/additional vehicle

ELEVATION: 7,250'

WHEELCHAIR ACCESS: Sites 1, 4, 6, 10, 16, 18, 19, 24, and 31; all group sites; restrooms

---

RESTRICTIONS:

PETS: Prohibited

FIRES: In fire rings only

ALCOHOL: Permitted

VEHICLES: Up to 25 feet

OTHER: 7-day stay limit, 2-day minimum stay on weekends; maximum 8 people/site (single), 16 people/site (double), 25 people/site (group sites A–C), or 50 people/site (group site D); gates locked 10 p.m.–7 a.m.

---

between the generously spaced campsites (with a few exceptions), so you'll be shielded from your many neighbors in this large campground. And although RVs are allowed, many RVers shy away from this campground because each site varies so dramatically in the size of RV it can accommodate.

Note: Like Redman Campground (see previous profile), Tanners Flat lies within Little Cottonwood Canyon, a protected watershed. Pets are prohibited here.

The campsites here are easy to access. Upon entering the campground and passing the host's gatehouse, sites 1–19 are to the right down closer to the trout-stocked river, and 20–36 climb to the left. The road throughout the entire campground is paved, including the parking spurs for each campsite. The sites themselves are a bit on the small side, but you'll have just enough room to set up your tent and unpack the car. The only inconvenience is the placement of toilet facilities, which are grouped near the north end of the campground. The only time you'll really notice, however, is if you're camping on that southern loop and you drank a little too much soda before bedtime.

Sites nearest the entrance will naturally have more vehicle and foot traffic; sites 4, 8–10, 13–15, and 18 have pull-through loops instead of parking spurs, which will attract more RVs. Try staying at the far end of the upper section in sites 32–36 to avoid crowds. Sites 3–6 will also keep you farther from the busy sections of the campground.

From Tanners Flat, you can jump off to one of several hikes in this popular canyon of the Wasatch Mountain Range. About a mile and a half farther up UT 210, you'll find the White Pine Trail. Shortly after this trail begins, it passes through an awesome visual reminder of the raw power of an avalanche: in the winter of 2004–05, tons of tumbling snow came down the mountain across the White Pine Trail, knocking down everything in its path. Today, the scar and the few lingering trees remain as a fascinating photo opportunity and chilling reminder.

If you've procrastinated deciding on a final destination for your hike, you'll have to make up your mind about a mile after the trailhead. The road forks at White Pine Fork Creek. Switchback left to go to White Pine Lake, or cross the creek right for Red Pine Lake. White Pine Lake is the longer hike at 9 miles round-trip; Red Pine Lake is steeper but only 6 miles round-trip. Both are pleasant alpine lakes that are worth the 2,000-foot climb. If you want more lake for your buck, then go to Red Pine and keep climbing to Upper Red Pine Lake and the surrounding ponds. Both lakes are stocked with feisty cutthroat trout that actually grow to a respectable size.

Farther up Little Cottonwood Canyon are more hiking opportunities: Hidden Peak, Maybird Gulch, Temple Quarry Nature Trail, and those near Albion Basin Campground (see page 12), to name a few. For detailed information about each hike, including length, altitude gain, difficulty, and description, go to www.fs.usda.gov/uwcnf and click "Recreation"; then click "Hiking" to access separate lists of overnight and day hikes in each ranger district.

It's easy to get caught up in planning far-off and exotic camping adventures, but sometimes it's nice to slip away for a night or two without much thought. In those times, there's no better campground than Tanners Flat.

Tanners Flat Campground

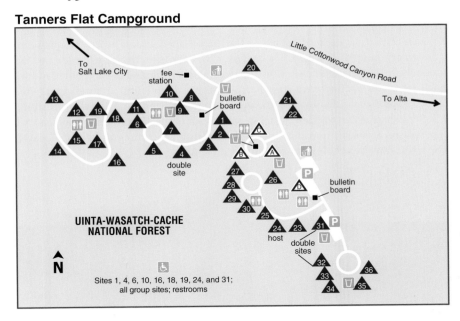

GETTING THERE

From the intersection of South 1300 East and UT 209 (East 9400 South) in Sandy, take UT 209 east 4.4 miles; then merge onto UT 210 (Little Cottonwood Canyon Road), proceed east another 4.1 miles up the canyon, and turn right onto Forest Road 220 to reach the campground.

GPS COORDINATES: N40° 34.316' W111° 42.041'

24

Timpooneke Campground

Beauty: ★★★★★ / Privacy: ★★★ / Quiet: ★★★ / Spaciousness: ★★★ / Security: ★★★★ / Cleanliness: ★★★★

Mount Timpanogos is an awesome sight, and Timpooneke Campground is the best seat in the house.

They say that if you look at the profile along the peaks of Mount Timpanogos, you'll see the outline of a young Native American princess lying down in peaceful rest. Some people look at Timpanogos as the home of Utah's very own glacier. Still others see the rugged mountain as the home of one of Utah's most talked-about hikes. No matter your angle, Mount Timpanogos is an awesome sight, and Timpooneke is the best seat in the house.

Timpooneke Campground is less than 10 miles from the Utah Valley, one of the fastest-growing parts of the state. The increased population here has had a corresponding effect on the tent-camping population at Timpooneke. Once a hidden gem that hardly anyone knew about, Timpooneke has been discovered, and reservations are almost a must these days. That's not to say that the campground isn't worth a visit or that you can't have privacy—you just have to be smart about picking your site.

Because the sites are spread out over a uniquely shaped layout, peace and quiet are still available to campers in the know. For starters, stay away from the loop located just before Timpooneke Road. These nine sites (6–14) are practically pinned to each other and would probably leave you wishing you'd stayed at another site. If you must choose a spot here, site 6, 7, or 12 here is passable. If you're staying over the weekend, you'll be a bit frustrated in sites 3–5—they're accessed from the main parking lot of the Timpooneke Trailhead, which fills up early on Saturday mornings and has cars constantly coming and going all day. During the week, however, these sites are actually quite nice.

Tibble Fork Reservoir

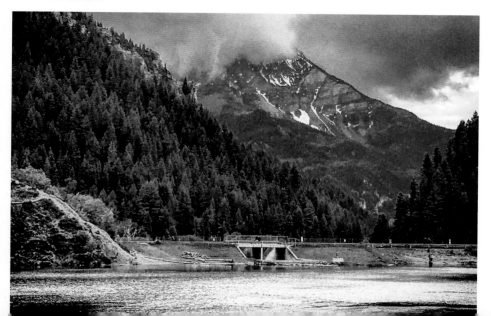

KEY INFORMATION

LOCATION: FR 056 south of UT 92, Provo, UT 84062

CONTACTS: 801-785-3563, tinyurl.com /uwcnfcamping; reservations: 877-444-6777, recreation.gov

OPERATED BY: American Land & Leisure for Uinta-Wasatch-Cache National Forest, Pleasant Grove Ranger District

OPEN: June–September (depending on weather)

SITES: 29 (including 7 doubles), plus 1 group site

EACH SITE: Picnic table, fire ring

ASSIGNMENT: First-come, first-served and by reservation

REGISTRATION: On-site self-registration or online

AMENITIES: Vault toilets, drinking water

PARKING: At campsites only

FEES: $21/night (single), $42/night (double), $100/night (group), $8/extra vehicle; $6 day-use fee

WHEELCHAIR ACCESS: All sites and restrooms

ELEVATION: 7,300'

RESTRICTIONS:

PETS: On leash only

FIRES: In fire rings only

ALCOHOL: Permitted

VEHICLES: 15- to 30-foot length limit

OTHER: 7-day stay limit; maximum 8 people /site (single), 16 people/site (double), or 40 people/site (group); gates locked 10 p.m.–7 a.m.

Your best bet for a high-quality camping experience enhanced by stunning views of the dramatic slopes of Timpanogos is on the back loop of the campground, in sites 15–30. The jewels here are sites 29 and 30, which don't have the views of the lower numbered sites but are tucked back on their own little dirt driveway spur just above the main road.

You'll usually be greeted at each campsite with perky little alpine wildflowers that put on a dazzling display during July; early in the year, you may also be greeted by patches of snow. The camp is always scheduled to open on Memorial Day weekend, but the camp host recommends not making any definite plans until later in June, depending on the severity of the previous winter. Bugs greet every camper at every site. Flies are always around, and mosquitoes vary year to year from thick to dense, buzzing clouds.

Despite its newfound popularity and permanent pest population, Timpooneke oozes charm. You'll wind along the Alpine Loop and see the canyon open up to stellar views of the valley below. In the fall, the road is full of Sunday drivers all week long, cruising for a chance to look at the brightly colored leaves. A small stream that runs through the upper loop of the campground looks like it comes straight from the snow-covered peaks above with the sole mission of gurgling for campground residents.

According to one version of the legend that named Mount Timpanogos, a young Native American princess named Ucanogas fell in love with Timpanac, a stranger from another tribe, when he came to her father in search of food. Their love ended in tragedy when jealous braves from Ucanogas's own tribe killed Timpanac by throwing him off the mountain peak during a challenge the chief had created to award his daughter's hand in marriage. Devastated, the princess died of a broken heart and was buried on top of the mountain, her silhouette still discernible.

The same challenges issued to Ucanogas's would-be suitors—running around a lake, hunting an animal, climbing a mountain peak—are some of the main attractions of Mount

Timpanogos today. American Fork Canyon has several lakes that are accessible to anglers. Try Tibble Fork Reservoir by heading 20 minutes back down the canyon and taking the fork on UT 144. This little reservoir is stocked with catchable rainbow trout that really come alive before dusk. Take the dirt road from Granite Flat Campground (located just above Tibble Fork Reservoir) to reach Silver Lake—a quieter, more challenging reservoir.

While you may not intend to hunt any animals, you'll at least see your fair share of them. Rocky Mountain goats, mule deer, moose, elk, and chipmunks are abundant in the 10,000-acre wilderness. There's also chance of seeing mountain lions or black bears, so follow safe backcountry protocol.

If you've got a hankering to climb a tall mountain peak, "Timp" is the hike to do. There are two routes to the summit: the Timpooneke Trail, an 18-mile round-trip journey, and the Aspen Grove Trail, a 16-mile jaunt along much of the same trail. It has been suggested, however, that the generally accepted mileage overestimates the actual distance. Mileage notwithstanding, you'll gain nearly 5,000 feet in elevation, and either hike will take you the better part of the day; also be mindful of rapidly changing weather. If you're not up for a long haul, try the easy footpath to Timpanogos Cave National Monument, a large cavern near the mouth of American Fork Canyon. All three hikes are featured in *60 Hikes Within 60 Miles: Salt Lake City,* by Greg Witt (Menasha Ridge Press).

Timpooneke Campground

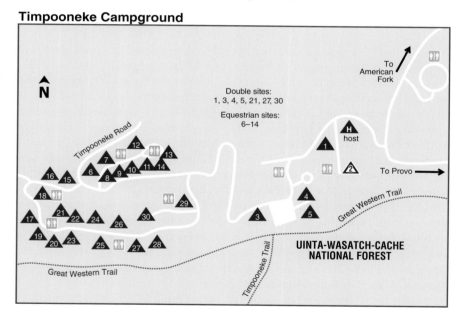

GETTING THERE

From I-15, take Exit 284 in Lehi (about 25 miles south of downtown Salt Lake City), and drive east on UT 92, which becomes the Alpine Loop Scenic Byway. In 15.7 miles, turn right at the T onto Forest Road 056, and drive another 0.7 mile to the campground.

GPS COORDINATES: N40° 26.016' W111° 38.184'

25

Tony Grove Campground

Beauty: ★★★★★ / Privacy: ★★★★ / Quiet: ★★★ / Spaciousness: ★★★★ / Security: ★★★★ /
Cleanliness: ★★★★

A good hike, a little fishing, a great campsite—what more could you ask for?

Tony Grove is the all-American campground. This sizable but tidy location has it all: a nearby lake full of lively fish, entrance to a fantastic trail system that leads to lakes and wilderness, easy access, and great campsites with plenty of room to set out your stuff.

Set deep in Uinta-Wasatch-Cache National Forest off US 89, this perfect little playground at 8,000 feet does everything right. You'll wander up the Logan Canyon Scenic Byway and turn off onto Forest Road 003. As the road weaves its way up to Tony Grove, you pass through the lower canyon brush and then stands of aspens that finally give way to spruce, pine, and fir. The drive alone is worth the trip, destination notwithstanding.

Don't misunderstand—here it's about the journey *and* the destination. As FR 003 ends, it gently delivers drivers into the small valley where Tony Grove Lake is located. At 25 acres, the lake is big enough to host more than a couple of canoes but not big enough to be intimidating.

The campground is located on the lake's southeastern shore, accessed by following the short driveway from FR 003. For the most part, the campground is a large loop with a small tail at the entrance. Stay on the backside of the loop—sites 10–23-ish—if you want to avoid a lot of foot traffic. Site 13 is off on its own, but you must climb a small stairway to reach it. Sites 29–31 offer the best access to the lake, although human nature indicates that you may

Looking across Tony Grove Lake to the northwestern shore

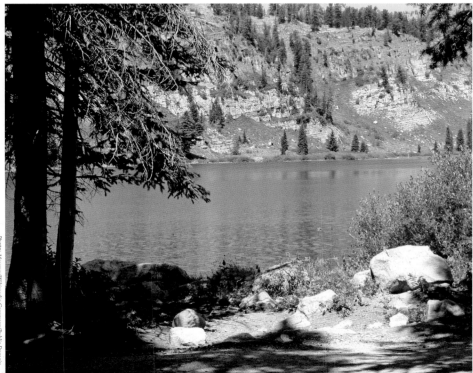

Photo: *Maserry/Wikimedia Commons/Public Domain*

KEY INFORMATION

LOCATION: FR 003 west of US 89, Logan, UT 84321

CONTACTS: 435-755-3620, tinyurl.com /uwcnfcamping; reservations: 877-444-6777 or recreation.gov

OPERATED BY: American Land & Leisure for Uinta-Wasatch-Cache National Forest, Logan Ranger District

OPEN: July–October

SITES: 36 (including 1 double)

EACH SITE: Picnic table, fire ring

ASSIGNMENT: First-come, first-served or by reservation (recommended)

REGISTRATION: On-site self-registration or online

AMENITIES: Vault toilets, drinking water, garbage service

PARKING: At campsites only

FEES: $19/night (single), $38/night (double), $8/extra vehicle; day use $6/day, $20/week, or $35/per season

WHEELCHAIR ACCESS: Sites 16b, 17b, and 18b

ELEVATION: 8,037'

RESTRICTIONS:

PETS: On leash only

FIRES: In fire rings only

ALCOHOL: Permitted

VEHICLES: Up to 30 feet

OTHER: 7-day stay limit; maximum 8 people/ site (single) or 16 people/site (double)

---

have people traipsing through your campsite on their way to and from the lake. After the turn, sites 32–37 are perched somewhat on a hill but are still accessible.

Sites here are generally well spaced and well proportioned. That extra space helps numb your brain to the fact that the campground is almost always full—you won't forget that fact, but you certainly won't feel like you're camping among 200 strangers. Because of high demand, many sites can be reserved. If you plan on showing up later than noon on a weekend, book ahead of time. If not, you're rolling the dice with the 23 first-come, first-served sites.

Bring your hiking boots to Tony Grove and try the hike to White Pine Lake. You gain a modest 1,250 feet of elevation over a 3.5-mile (one-way) trip, which ends at lovely White Pine Lake, between Mounts Gog and Magog less than 0.5 mile from the Mount Naomi Wilderness boundary.

The daily pay-parking lot also hosts the trailhead to Naomi Peak. This trail requires a little more exertion out of its hikers, topping out at just below 10,000 feet. Try to plan your hike in late July or early August, and you'll be treated to a feast of wildflower colors on an alpine platter. You'll also be rewarded with views of several deep canyons that claw their way toward the peak in a sensational and sometimes eerily shadowed fashion.

Longer hikes to Green Canyon and High Creek funnel out to Cache Valley on the other side of the mountain. Hiked in reverse, this would be a great alternative to taking the paved roads to Tony Grove. Let a lesser outdoorsman take the car—you can hike the 10 or 15 miles from Cache Valley! If you happen to be the lesser outdoorsman (or if you're just not crazy), take one of the shorter hikes. An interpretive nature trail near the lake is made especially for sauntering.

Pack your fishing pole and try the action at Tony Grove Lake. It's fished heavily but stocked regularly, so you have a decent chance at catching your dinner—though you probably won't pull a trophy from these waters.

The Logan River is a more highly prized fishery. Anywhere along US 89 should yield a day of challenging but memorable angling. Other small creeks in the area are hit-and-miss, but those can sometimes be the most rewarding experiences: miss . . . miss . . . *hit*!

If you have a canoe, kayak, raft, or inner tube, this is the place to bring it. Tony Grove Lake's frigid waters take some getting used to, but a quick dip is just what the doctor ordered on a sunny summer afternoon. Paddle across the lake to get a better view of the cliffs that seem to hover over the lake as bodyguards.

It's a shame that Tony Grove is open for only a few months each summer. (The snow-mobiling crowd is fond of it in the winter, but it's just not the same.) A good hike, a little fishing, a great campsite—what more could you ask for?

Tony Grove Campground

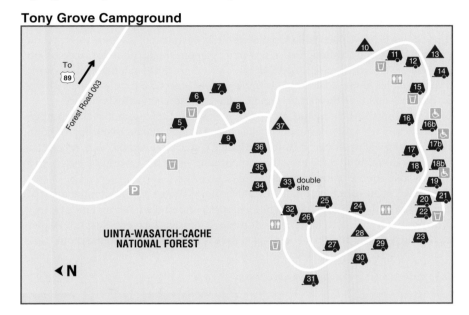

GETTING THERE

From the intersection of US 91 (Main Street) and US 89 (East 400 North) in Logan, drive 21.7 miles east on US 89. Turn left onto FR 141 and then make another quick left onto FR 003, heading south and then west. In 6.7 miles, turn left to enter the campground.

GPS COORDINATES: N41° 53.633' W111° 38.393'

26

⚠️ Yellowpine Campground

Beauty: ★★★★ / Privacy: ★★★ / Quiet: ★★★★ / Spaciousness: ★★★★ / Security: ★★★★ /
Cleanliness: ★★★★

This campground is functional and friendly to campers of all levels of ability.

Yellow pine is the common name for ponderosa pine (*Pinus ponderosa*). Look around at Yellowpine Campground, and you'll find plenty of living specimens of this fantastic forest resident. Ponderosa pines, lodgepole pines, and aspens fill the campground. When a lofty alpine breeze makes its way up the canyon, it rustles the trees' high crowns to create a whispery and enchanting song.

Tucked just below Upper Stillwater Reservoir in the midst of all these trees, Yellowpine Campground has one attribute that so few other campgrounds can boast: accessibility. I'm not just talking about the paved road that takes you there (although that sinuous stretch of road that rambles along Rock Creek is undoubtedly accessible to any driver); I'm talking about the accessibility of the campground facilities to campers with disabilities.

The U.S. Forest Service has put forth an obvious effort to ensure that this campground is functional and friendly to campers of all levels of ability. The entire campground loop is paved, as are the walkways to and from each paved picnic table and fire ring. A paved nature trail and wooden fishing dock near the campground open up a world of possibilities not always available at other campgrounds.

Be careful when searching out Yellowpine online. There's a campground along Mirror Lake Highway in Uinta-Wasatch-Cache National Forest called Yellow Pine (two words), and mixing them up could leave invited guests confused. Incidentally, both Ashley and Uinta-Wasatch-Cache National Forests also have a Willows Campground, both Dixie and

The campground road, dressed up in autumn finery

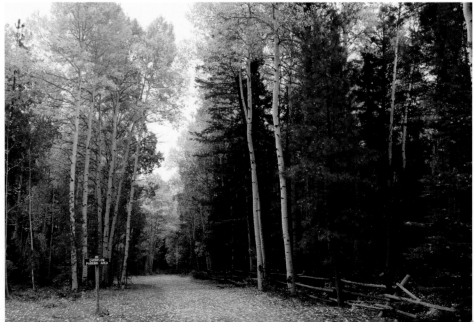

Photo: Sheila Harper/U.S. Forest Service

KEY INFORMATION

LOCATION: FR 134, Duchesne, UT 84021

CONTACTS: 435-738-2482, tinyurl.com /ashleynfcamping; reservations: 877-444-6777, recreation.gov

OPERATED BY: Ashley National Forest, Duchesne/Roosevelt Ranger District

OPEN: May–September

SITES: 29 (includes 4 doubles), plus 2 group sites

EACH SITE: Picnic table, fire ring

ASSIGNMENT: Sites 18–29 first-come, first-served; sites 1–17 and group sites by reservation

REGISTRATION: On-site self-registration or online

AMENITIES: Restrooms, drinking water, garbage service

PARKING: At campsites only

FEES: $10/night (single), $16/night (double), $30/night (group)

WHEELCHAIR ACCESS: All sites and restrooms

ELEVATION: 7,601'

RESTRICTIONS:

PETS: On leash only

FIRES: In fire rings only

ALCOHOL: Permitted

VEHICLES: Up to 30 feet

OTHER: 14-day stay limit; maximum 8 people/site (single), 16 people/site (double), or 32 people/site (group)

Uinta-Wasatch-Catche have a Spruces Campground, and Ponderosa Campground (page 72) shares a name with a group campground along Mirror Lake Highway. When you invite friends to meet you at camp, be specific!

Before you go thinking the entire place looks more like a paved supermarket parking lot than a campground, take into account the efforts of Mother Nature to provide a real outdoors experience. The massive trees make such little pavement look inconsequential, so you really don't much notice the asphalt beneath you.

One of the best ways to identify ponderosa and lodgepole pines is by their tall, straight trunks—lodgepoles more so than ponderosas. They typically have fewer branches near the ground, which means that campsites here aren't as private as they might be in the presence of, say, firs or cedars. That's OK, though—you'll find enough privacy to be comfortable.

Both species of trees have been an important part of Utah's history. Lodgepoles, found primarily here in the Uintas, were used extensively in the state's early years for railroad ties and as poles for fences; they're still used as lumber for construction. Ponderosas are a highly utilized timber for mill products today, just as they were in the days when Utah was being settled. Before that time, the Nez Perce and Crow used the pitch for glue, and the Cheyenne applied it to the inside of their flutes to improve the sound.

The first 17 sites on the loop can be reserved online; the remaining 12 are first-come, first-served. You'll probably want to book well in advance, although I was surprised on my visit to see only a handful of spots taken. Then again, that's the beauty of showing up on a Thursday afternoon.

Rock Creek itself provides pretty good fishing opportunities, rainbows and browns mostly. There are even a few good pools on the South Fork of Rock Creek as it enters Rock Creek proper, but only for a mile or so. The upper reaches of the South Fork are gorgeous but devoid of fish—probably due to natural barriers in the river created by avalanches and a steep riverbed.

Don't let the lack of fish discourage you from taking the dirt road up the South Fork. The river is gorgeous up this high and a pleasure just to view. From just below Upper Stillwater Campground, take Forest Road 134 to its fork with FR 135 and then stay right at the junction, which puts you on FR 143. FR 143 follows the South Fork and eventually plants you at a vague trail to Arta and Survey Lakes. (These are both planted with small trout, although the fish are often casualties of severe winters.) The hike is short but steep to both lakes.

FR 135 actually takes you over the mountain and back down again before it reconnects with UT 35 near Hannah. If you're looking for a different way home or a scenic drive, this is an excellent choice. There's even a brief Bryce Canyon–esque feel to the cliffs on the north side of the mountain ridge, where a jagged outcropping of spires clings to the solid cliff wall behind it. It's a magnificent route, but it does require a high-clearance vehicle.

You don't have to be a dendrologist (tree geek) to enjoy Yellowpine. In fact, that's what makes it so valuable—it can be enjoyed by many people for many different reasons.

Yellowpine Campground

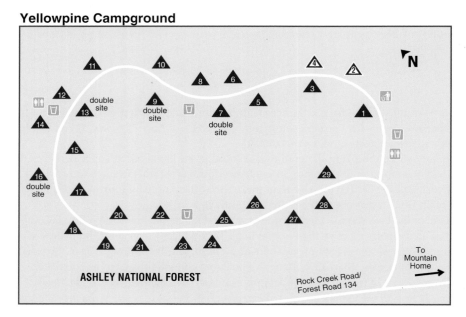

GETTING THERE

From the intersection of US 40 (Main Street) and UT 87 (North Center Street) in the town of Duchesne, drive north on UT 87 and, in 5.9 miles, turn left (northwest) onto UT 35. In 3.4 miles, turn right (northwest) onto Rock Creek Road. In 16.4 miles, turn right at the T and then make a quick jog left to continue northwest on Rock Creek Road, which becomes Forest Road 134. In 8.4 miles, look for the turnoff to the campground on your right.

GPS COORDINATES: N40° 32.131' W110° 38.261'

WESTERN UTAH

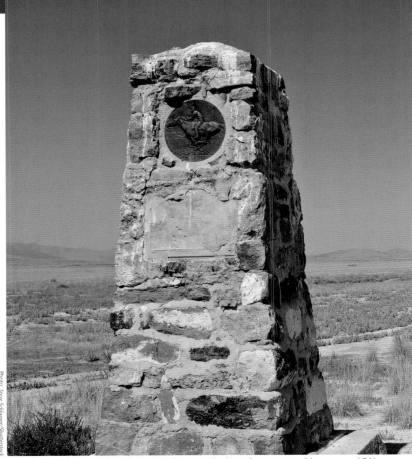

Pony Express historical marker near Simpson Springs Campground (see page 101)

27

Clear Creek Campground

Beauty: ★★★ / Privacy: ★★★★★ / Quiet: ★★★★★ / Spaciousness: ★★★★ / Security: ★★★★★ /
Cleanliness: ★★★★

Solitude exists in spades in this cozy little campground.

Pop quiz: How many national forests are there in Utah? Five? Wrong. Six? Nope. Try seven. Avid outdoorsmen could probably rattle off the first five: Ashley, Dixie, Fishlake, Manti–La Sal, and Uinta-Wasatch-Cache. But Caribou-Targhee and Sawtooth? Yep. And Sawtooth holds one of Utah's sweet little treasures—Clear Creek Campground.

Like an island surrounded by a sea of unremarkable countryside, the Raft River Mountain Range in Sawtooth National Forest is all alone in northwestern Utah. If being all alone doesn't sound so bad, then make Clear Creek Campground the top priority on your to-camp list. Solitude exists in spades in this cozy little campground.

Clear Creek is truly isolated. There's no fee, there are no numbers on the campsites, and there's not much indication that more than a handful of people ever make it here, especially on a weekday. Don't mistake isolation for desolation, though. The campground's namesake, sparkling Clear Creek, makes its way through the camp and gives life to numerous tall aspens and evergreens, with a healthy riparian understory of thick brush along the creek's shores

The Bull Flat Trail heads southwest from the campground.

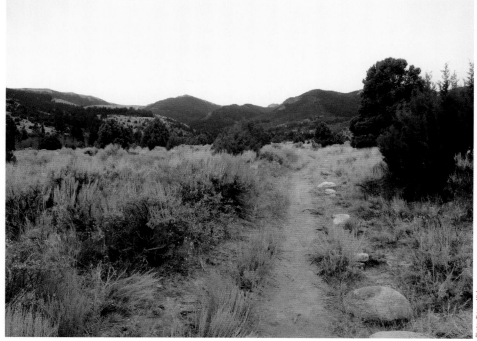

Photo: Tristan Higbee

KEY INFORMATION

ADDRESS: FR 001, Malta, UT 83342

CONTACT: 208-678-0430, tinyurl.com
/sawtoothnfcamping

OPERATED BY: Sawtooth National Forest,
Minidoka Ranger District

OPEN: June–September

SITES: 8, according to my count

EACH SITE: Picnic table, fire ring

ASSIGNMENT: First-come, first-served;
no reservations

REGISTRATION: None

FACILITIES: Vault toilets

PARKING: At campsites only

FEE: None

WHEELCHAIR ACCESS: All sites

ELEVATION: 6,303'

RESTRICTIONS:

PETS: On leash only

FIRES: In fire rings only

ALCOHOL: Permitted

VEHICLES: Up to 30 feet

OTHER: 14-day stay limit; 2 vehicles/site;
horses prohibited

and throughout the camp's gentle hillside. The creek is also rumored to hold small trout for sneak-attack-style fishing, although someone must have given them warning when I came— I've never actually seen any myself.

The campsites here are mostly unremarkable, each with a small fire pit and picnic table on a flat patch of ground; they're not numbered at the campground, but I've labeled them on the map here for reference. You shouldn't have any trouble snagging site 7 or 8 to maximize privacy if there are other campers around. Sites 1 and 2 should be your last pick. Their lack of shade and exposure to the road make them less desirable than others farther down the road. The U.S. Forest Service says there are 12 sites total, but I found only 8. Perhaps the other 4 were hiding with the fish?

Even though the driving directions on the next page may sound a bit convoluted, getting to the campground is actually easy. Don't panic when you see the WELCOME TO IDAHO signs on UT 42—you'll briefly enter the Gem State before dipping back into Utah by following the brown recreation signs. The family car will make the well-maintained dirt road just fine, but bring plenty of supplies. Snowville (population 177) is the closest sign of civilization, but you'll have to make it to Brigham City, Utah, or Burley, Idaho, for real supplies. Each is somewhere on the order of an hour and a half away, each way.

There's lots of exploring to be done in the Raft River Range. Most notable are hikes from the Bull Flat Trailhead, approximately across from what I have labeled as site 5 on the map, just before the back loop of the campground. Take a fork off the main trail after about a mile to go to Bull Flat, or stay on the main trail to climb to beautiful Bull Lake, and then on to the peak of Bull Mountain. Once atop the summit, you'll have staggering views of Utah, Idaho, and Nevada. With the campground at a little more than 6,300 feet in elevation and the peak at just less than 10,000, you should be prepared to climb. Take the trail as an overnight backpacking trip to help break up all the steep terrain and give you more time to see the sights.

On the other side of the mountain you may notice a large, cavelike opening etched out of the stone face high on the hilltop. I wouldn't recommend making the trek up there; there's no real trail to the area, and it's incredibly steep and rugged. There are, however, remnants of a few old mines if you decide to head off in that direction. Do so at your own risk, and be aware and respectful of the plentiful fences and private property boundaries in the area.

Once you've discovered the Raft River Range, you'll likely want to come back again and again. The Clear Creek and Bull Flat areas only hold a portion of the surprises you might find in this unique little mountain range. Its western reaches also have little canyons with spring-fed streams folded inside.

If you didn't pass the pop quiz, here's your chance to take a field trip to Sawtooth National Forest. Coincidentally, the other seldom-known national forest in Utah, Caribou-Targhee, occupies only a small dot of Utah turf on the Box Elder–Cache county line. There are no formal campgrounds there, but Clarkston Mountain's Gunsight Peak looms at 8,244 feet.

Sawtooth may not be the biggest or most famous of Utah national forests, but it holds hidden treasures for the solitude seekers willing to find them.

Clear Creek Campground

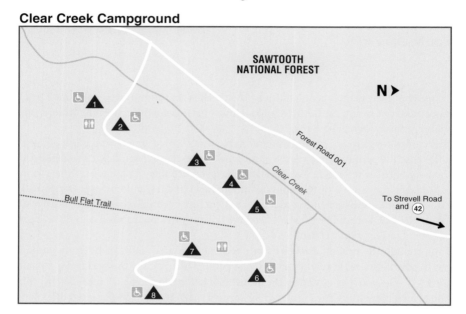

GETTING THERE

From I-84, take Exit 5 in Snowville (about 108 miles northwest of Salt Lake City) and head west on UT 30. In 15.6 miles, the road forks—where UT 30 heads left, keep straight (north) to continue on UT 42 into Idaho; at the state line, UT 42 becomes ID 81. In 8.6 miles, turn left (west) onto Strevell Road. After 3 miles, turn left (south) onto Clear Creek Road (Forest Road 001) to head back into Utah. In 2.8 miles, bear right at the fork to continue on Clear Creek Road, and drive another 3.2 miles to the campground entrance, on your left.

GPS COORDINATES: N41° 57.214' W113° 19.381'

Clover Spring Campground

Beauty: ★★★ / Privacy: ★★★ / Quiet: ★★★ / Spaciousness: ★★★★ / Security: ★★★★ / Cleanliness: ★★★★

It's almost hypnotic to stand near the bubbling water.

The Goshute tribe named it Shambip, early settlers regarded it as their lifeblood, and members of the Civilian Conservation Corps (CCC) once called it home. Although now it's just known as Clover Spring Campground, it's still relatively unknown, and a neat little place to spend the night in your tent.

Because it's just 60 miles from Salt Lake City, you'd expect this 11-site campground to fill up every night with urbanites looking for a quick overnight getaway. On the contrary, that demographic seems to congregate in the canyons of the Wasatch Front, leaving Clover Spring to the locals and the lucky few who have discovered its location.

The campground has two sections: sites 1–7, where horses are prohibited, and sites 8–11, where they're welcome. Upon entering the campground, the division of these two factions is apparent; equestrians go right along a gentle incline to find large hitching rails and watering troughs, and the horseless go left to choose from several sites that sit along the shores of Clover Creek.

Snag site 2, 4, or 6 for the most shade and privacy. You'll also have the bonus of being sung to sleep at night by the icy-cold waters of Clover Creek, which flow just feet from each of these sites. The creek is actually born right here in the campground at the springs, which lie just up from site 2. It's almost hypnotic to stand near the bubbling water as it burps out of the ground and flows away.

Retro-looking BLM signage points the way into the campground.

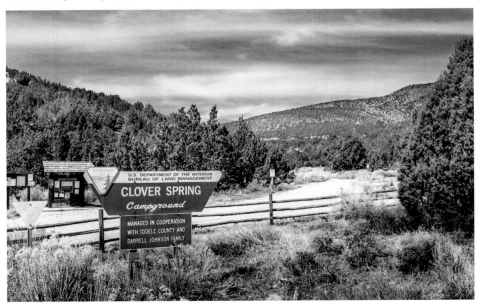

KEY INFORMATION

LOCATION: UT 199, Rush Valley, UT 84069

CONTACT: 801-977-4300, blm.gov/utah

OPERATED BY: Bureau of Land Management, Salt Lake Field Office

OPEN: May–November (depending on weather)

SITES: 10, plus 1 group site

EACH SITE: Picnic table, fire ring

ASSIGNMENT: First-come, first-served; group site reservable by calling the number above

REGISTRATION: On-site self-registration

AMENITIES: Vault toilets

PARKING: At campsites only

FEES: $12/night (single), $45/night (group)

WHEELCHAIR ACCESS: Not designated

ELEVATION: 6,004'

RESTRICTIONS:

PETS: Permitted

ALCOHOL: Permitted

FIRES: In fire rings only

VEHICLES: Up to 30 feet

OTHER: 14-day stay limit; maximum 8 people, 2 vehicles/site (single) or 50 people, 10 vehicles/site (group); shooting and off-road vehicles prohibited. The campground abuts private property, so heed posted NO TRESPASSING signs.

The springs have given life to towering cottonwood trees and green grasses in the campsites closest to the water. This burst of green fades into hardy junipers that dot the entire hillside here at the base of the Onaqui Mountains.

The equestrian side is decidedly less lush, being removed from the water. If all the lower sites are taken, sites 10 and 11 are actually quite nice, and you won't see much traffic up there at the end of the campground road. They slip under juniper cover and are quite cozy in their own right.

Site 7 is also worthy of consideration as a group site. It's got ample parking, plenty of shade, and enough seating and serving areas to keep it from feeling crowded. At $45 per night, it's the only site in the campground that can be reserved.

You may be tempted to cup your hands in the waters of Clover Spring and gulp down the spring water, especially in the summer months when this campground sizzles, but campers are warned not to drink the water. Also, the toilets are only small huts, and although they're tidy and functional, you'll definitely know you've left the comforts of home.

In 2017, a camper posting to an unofficial Clover Spring Facebook page reported a mountain lion sighting here. Her dogs sent the cougar packing, but see page 5 for what to do in case of a more prolonged encounter.

Horseback riding is one of the big draws to Clover Spring, but don't feel that you can't explore using your own two legs. The Onaqui Range is more hills than mountains, but it still holds days and days full of exploration. Find seasonal springs, old mines, and cute little canyons littering the range. Flowering cacti dot the landscape, and even the occasional sego lily, Utah's state flower, can be found and photographed. The range tops out at around 9,000 feet for climbers adamant about finding the best views. Trails are sketchy, but a small trail that introduces you to the area leaves right from camp.

Continue up UT 199 to Fisher Pass (shown on most maps as Johnson Pass, but on-site signs all read Fisher) for some great views of Utah's West Desert to the west and the Oquirrh Mountains back to the east. This area was once buzzing with activity in the mid-1930s as members of the CCC's Company 2517 worked in the area and were based where the campground now sits. Imagine what these young men might have thought, many of them from the more rain-blessed regions of the eastern United States, as they looked out over Fisher Pass to Utah's most desolate region.

The Onaqui Mountains are sandwiched between two pockets of national-forest land: the Deseret Peak complex to the north and the Sheeprock Mountains/Vernon Reservoir complex to the south. Deseret Peak is discussed in the profile for Loop Campground (see next page). To explore the Sheeprock area, head back out to UT 36 and drive south to Vernon. Follow the signs just past town to Vernon Reservoir, and you'll have access to several dirt roads that wind around those hills.

Clover Spring is open through November, weather permitting. By this time, most other campgrounds in northern Utah are closed, so this is an ideal place to keep in your back pocket for those times in late fall when you're itching to get out but you don't have the time to travel to southern Utah. If spring weather has been cooperative, the sites here may be campable earlier than May.

Clover Spring Campground

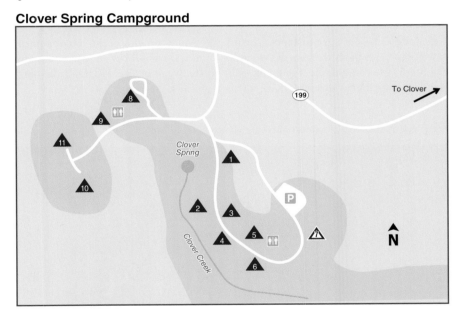

GETTING THERE

From the intersection of UT 36 and UT 112 in Tooele, go 17 miles south on UT 36; then turn right onto UT 199. Continue 7.9 miles west to the campground entrance, on your left.

GPS COORDINATES: N40° 20.827' W112° 33.019'

29

Loop Campground

Beauty: ★★★★★ / Privacy: ★★★★ / Quiet: ★★★★ / Spaciousness: ★★★★ / Security: ★★★★ /
Cleanliness: ★★★★

Once you visit Loop Campground, you'll want to tell everyone about the Stansbury Mountains.

The lonely Stansbury Mountains can make you feel like you're stranded on an island, but you should be so lucky to be stuck with this mountain range to explore. Surrounded by sand and sage on three sides and the Great Salt Lake to the northeast, the Stansbury Range is a bona fide oasis in the desert.

Six different campgrounds lie along South Willow Canyon Road, Loop being the last, abutting the Deseret Peak Wilderness. It lives up to its name: the long, skinny campground loop is created where the road turns to direct cars back down the canyon.

Along the loop are campsites that are average in size and in well-used condition. Within the loop is a smaller circular turnoff where you can access sites 3–5. If you can, pick another site besides these—site 1, for instance. The first site you'll come to, at the top of a steep dirt driveway, this is probably the gem of the campground. If you're lucky enough to snag it, you probably won't see another human being while you're in camp. Sites 1A and 2, the next two sites on the loop going clockwise, make for semi-shielded camping.

Looking up at the Stansbury Mountains from the campground

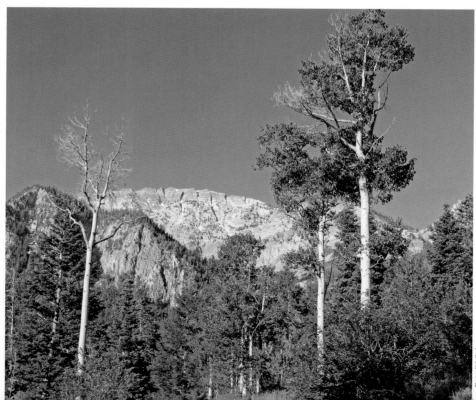

Photo: Kyle Dodson

KEY INFORMATION

LOCATION: South Willow Canyon Road, Dugway, UT 84022

CONTACT: 801-733-2660, tinyurl.com /uwcnfcamping

OPERATED BY: American Land & Leisure for Uinta-Wasatch-Cache National Forest, Salt Lake Ranger District

OPEN: Late May–mid-October (depending on weather)

SITES: 10 (including 1 double)

EACH SITE: Picnic table, fire ring

ASSIGNMENT: First-come-first served; no reservations

REGISTRATION: On-site self-registration

AMENITIES: Vault toilets

PARKING: At campsites and Mill Fork Trailhead

FEE: $14/night (single), $28/night (double), $8/additional vehicle

WHEELCHAIR ACCESS: Not designated

ELEVATION: 7,440'

RESTRICTIONS:

PETS: On leash only

FIRES: In fire rings only

ALCOHOL: Permitted

VEHICLES: RVs and trailers not recommended due to narrow access road

OTHER: 7-day stay limit; maximum 8 people/site (single) or 16 people/site (double)

The biggest disadvantage to camping at Loop is the lack of drinking water, although a nearby stream provides all the water you care to filter. Old but usable vault toilets are evenly spaced among the sites.

The main draws to this part of the Stansbury Range are the Deseret Peak Wilderness and the 4-mile (one-way) Mill Fork Trail to Deseret Peak. Loop Campground serves as the trailhead for the hike, so there's a small parking area at the top of the loop. If you're in good condition, get up early and hike to the peak. You'll have to make more than 3,500 feet in elevation, but the 360-degree views are unmatched. From Deseret Peak, look around and you'll see that in a way, you really are on an island. The Great Basin—miles and miles of nothing—surrounds you. Pack a lunch and enjoy your position on top of the desert while gazing at the rocky outcropping and patchwork of pine and aspen on the canyon floor. Just be sure to head down if there's any sign of a storm. Lightning and bald mountain peaks don't mix well for hikers; add in wet rocks on a steep trail, and you've got a recipe for one heck of a laceration cocktail.

The Deseret Peak hike isn't your only option in the 25,000-acre wilderness. Instead of staying on the Mill Fork Trail, you could take the Willow Lakes Trail, which clings to the hillside and skirts around a couple of valleys before dropping you into South Willow Lake. Climb back out and hug one more ridge to reach North Willow Lake. Just beware of so-called shortcuts—no matter how skilled you think you are, dropping down into one of these valleys to follow the river back to camp is a bad idea, especially in the snow . . . or so I've heard.

For some reason, Loop and the other campgrounds of South Willow Canyon aren't used nearly as much as the campgrounds in the Wasatch Range. Perhaps it's the old adage, "Out of sight, out of mind." The Oquirrh Mountains stand between the Salt Lake Valley and the Stansbury Mountains, blocking the latter from view in Utah's most populated area. Consequently, you've got a good chance of finding a site at Loop, even when campgrounds in the Big and Little Cottonwood Canyons of the Wasatch Range are bursting at the seams. The hiking trails here are also in better shape—less litter, fewer signs of human damage, and more solitude.

Don't mistake "forgotten" for "neglected," though. There is a small ranger station in the canyon, and the campgrounds are often patrolled. The dedication of the rangers ensures the protection of this precious and rare resource in the desert, but it also means that you need to make doubly sure you're familiar with forest and wilderness regulations before heading out. Mountain bikes and off-road vehicles are often seen in the canyon but are prohibited within the wilderness boundary.

Once you visit Loop Campground, you'll want to tell everyone about the Stansbury Mountains. Instead of just telling them, though, why not load them in the car and head out to the desert? Just when they think you've gone nuts, you'll make the turn into South Willow Canyon, leave the pavement, and crawl up to Loop. You'll open their eyes to a sweet little mountain retreat and have a quiet little piece of the "island" all to yourselves.

Loop Campground

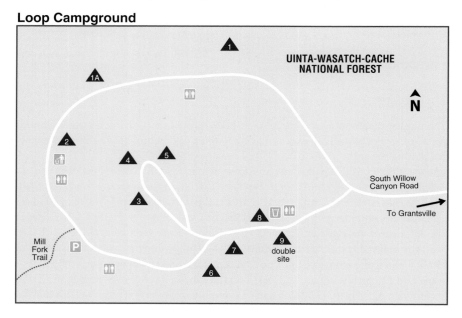

GETTING THERE

From downtown Salt Lake City west of I-15, take I-80 west 20 miles to Exit 99 (Lake Point/ UT 36). Go 3.5 miles south on UT 36; then turn right onto UT 138. After 10.9 miles, turn left onto South West Street in Grantsville, just after the brown sign on your right for North and South Willow Canyon Roads and Loop Campground. Drive south about 5 miles—West Street becomes Mormon Trail—and bear right at the fork onto South Willow Canyon Road (Forest Road 171), which changes from pavement to gravel. Loop Campground is 7 miles farther, at the turnaround for South Willow Canyon.

GPS COORDINATES: N40° 28.987′ W112° 36.386′

30

Simpson Springs Campground

Beauty: ★★★ / Privacy: ★★ / Quiet: ★★★★★ / Spaciousness: ★★★ / Security: ★★★★★ /
Cleanliness: ★★★★★

The West Desert is alive and rich with history, wildlife, and plenty for campers to do.

In the mid-1800s, a long-distance relationship would have been nearly impossible. It took six months to get a message from one end of the country to the other. That's an entire year from the time you asked, "Do you still love me?" and your sweetie replied, "Wait, who are you again?"

Three enterprising men set out to change that: W. H. Russell, Alexander Majors, and William B. Waddell. Their plan: set up a series of sprinting horses that could carry messages from coast to coast in just 10 days. On January 27, 1860, they announced the formation of the Pony Express.

Simpson Springs, in Utah's West Desert, was an important watering station and rest house for riders along the route. Although the Pony Express operated for less than two years, its heritage has been preserved at Simpson Springs.

A large campground just off the old Pony Express route is home to 20 smallish sites, each equipped with its own picnic table and not much else. Water is available from several spigots around the campground, but it must be treated before drinking.

So many buildings have been erected, destroyed, replaced, and repaired in the Simpson Springs area that no one is quite sure which building was the original Pony Express station. Today, a small reimagined station stands across the road from the campground as a re-creation of what the original building would have looked like, in what is believed to be

This replica of the Simpson Springs Pony Express station sits just across the road from the campground.

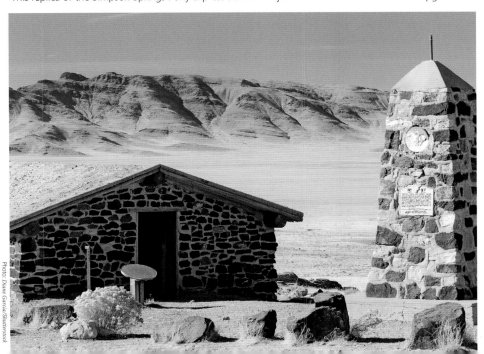

Photo: Diane Garcia/Shutterstock

KEY INFORMATION

LOCATION: Simpson Springs Road (Pony Express National Historic Trail), Vernon, UT 84080

CONTACT: 801-977-4300, blm.gov/utah

OPERATED BY: Bureau of Land Management, Salt Lake Field Office

OPEN: Year-round

SITES: 20

EACH SITE: Fire pits, picnic table, barbecue stand

ASSIGNMENT: First-come, first-served; no reservations

REGISTRATION: On-site self-registration

AMENITIES: Vault toilets, nonpotable water

PARKING: At campsites only

FEE: $15/night

WHEELCHAIR ACCESS: Not designated

ELEVATION: 4,890'

RESTRICTIONS:

PETS: Permitted

FIRES: In fire rings only

ALCOHOL: Permitted

VEHICLES: Up to 20 feet

OTHER: 14-day stay limit; maximum 8 people, 2 vehicles/site

the approximate place the original was built. Duck inside the squatty little cabin and try to imagine yourself being a pony rider coming in from his hot, dusty sprint for a little rest and shelter from the sun.

Several interpretive signs are located back toward the parking area, including a brief history that recounts the rise and fall of the Pony Express, as well as the chronicled history of Simpson Springs itself.

Summers can be scorching in the West Desert, so most people come to Simpson Springs in the cool seasons. If that's your plan, just make sure that it hasn't been too wet for the days preceding your trip; the dirt road can get a little slick. Otherwise, your family sedan will make the trip just fine.

If you must travel in summer, try to get site 1 or 20 for shade. In cooler weather, sites 8, 18, or 19 are set a bit back from the others to offer a bit of privacy (though not much) in an otherwise uncovered landscape.

The completion of the transcontinental telegraph line rendered the Pony Express obsolete, and the area lay largely unattended for 80 years, but Simpson Springs enjoyed a resurgence in the 1940s. From 1939 to 1942, the Civilian Conservation Corps (CCC) built barracks, a mess hall, a swimming pool, and other buildings as a base for its range and road operations in the valley. The development was torn down at the beginning of World War II, but its foundations and other remnants line the road up to the campground.

Simpson Springs also hosts a menagerie of Utah's most unique wildlife. Hundreds of pronghorn antelope live in the hills surrounding the old Pony Express Trail and cross the road each day as they graze in the area. Hawks rule the skies, and if you're really lucky, you may even catch a glimpse of one of the herds of wild horses in the region. The Bureau of Land Management (BLM) manages some 5,400 wild horses and 300 wild burros throughout Utah. I was lucky enough to see about a dozen of these magnificent creatures on my way to the campground. The Wild West indeed!

Continue west nearly 40 miles along the Pony Express Trail to visit Fish Springs National Wildlife Refuge, where you'll encounter a true oasis in the desert. Scores of birds, mammals, reptiles, and even a native fish call this 18,000-acre refuge (10,000-acre marsh) home. Pack your camera to take pictures of some of these species around the refuge; you'll probably need the photos to persuade your friends that this place really exists. See fws.gov/refuge/fish_springs for more information.

Another 40 miles to the west of Fish Springs are the Deep Creek Mountains, a sharp series of peaks that rise dramatically from the flat desert floor. Here, you'll find a few small creeks with beautifully colored small trout and a chance to hike the daunting 12,087-foot Ibapah Peak. Most hikers stay at the BLM's rustic CCC campground south of Callao. It's barely more than a scratch in the ground, but it will suffice. Day-trip from Simpson Springs if you don't mind the long drive—just be sure that no matter where you camp, you pack extra fuel. There are no gas stations for miles and miles and uninformed travelers have been known to run out of gas and walk for hours to find help.

Unbeknownst to most Utahns, the world doesn't end after the city of Tooele. The West Desert is alive and rich with history, wildlife, and plenty for campers to do; and there's no place better to start your discoveries than at Simpson Springs.

Simpson Springs Campground

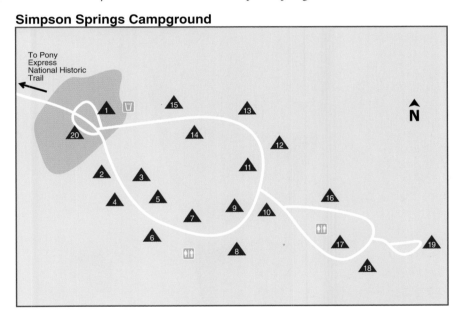

GETTING THERE

From the town of Vernon, head north on UT 36. About 5 miles north of the LDS church and Vernon Elementary School, turn left (west) onto the Pony Express National Historic Trail, also known here as Lookout Pass Road/Pony Express Road and farther west as Simpson Springs Road. After Lookout Pass, about 8 miles from UT 36, the road turns to dirt. About 13 miles from Lookout Pass, the road forks—bear left (south) and continue 3.5 miles to the campground entrance, on your left.

GPS COORDINATES: N40° 2.202' W112° 47.268'

SOUTHERN UTAH

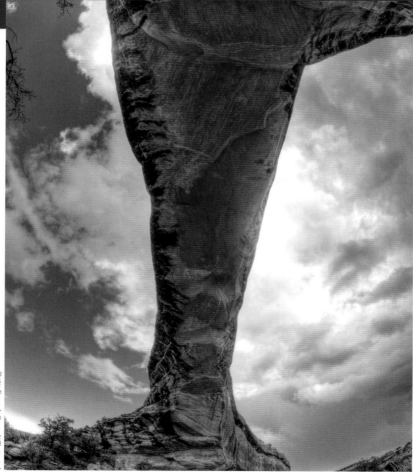

Photo: Tomasz L. Czarnecki/Shutterstock

Owachomo Bridge, Natural Bridges National Monument (see page 141)

31

⛺ Arches National Park:
HITTLE BOTTOM CAMPGROUND

Beauty: ★★★★★ / Privacy: ★★★★ / Quiet: ★★★★ / Spaciousness: ★★★★ / Security: ★★★★ /
Cleanliness: ★★★★

Enjoy the spectacular sights, from the verdant riparian riverway to the soaring sandstone spires.

Hittle Bottom Campground sits just 6 miles outside of the eastern edge of Arches National Park, but to get there you'll pass the turnoff to the park on US 191, turn up UT 128, and then drive 30 miles to reach it. As you make your way up the Colorado River on sinuous UT 128, enjoy the spectacular sights, from the verdant riparian riverway to the soaring sandstone spires. The drive is definitely worth it.

Hittle Bottom is a true hidden gem—far enough away from the bustle of Moab and Arches to give you a peaceful camping experience, yet close enough that you can access any of the area's main attractions with only a short commute.

Arches National Park is an obvious day-trip destination if you're based at Hittle Bottom. Though relatively small as national parks go, at just under 75,000 acres, it's unlike any other place on Earth in its concentration of naturally occurring arches. At last count, it held more than 2,000 named arch formations, with more likely to be discovered. These airy openings in otherwise-solid stone walls excite the imagination of park visitors and set the perfect backdrop frame for anyone who wants to take a photo.

Hittle Bottom is far enough from the park to give you solitude but close enough to be convenient.

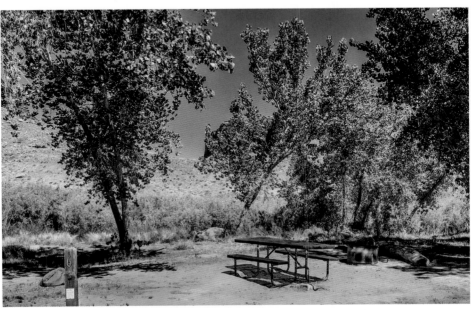

KEY INFORMATION

LOCATION: UT 128 northeast of Moab, UT 84532

CONTACTS: 435-259-2100, blm.gov/utah; reservations: 877-444-6777, recreation.gov

OPERATED BY: Bureau of Land Management, Moab Field Office

OPEN: Year-round

SITES: 14, plus 1 group site

EACH SITE: Picnic table, metal fire ring

ASSIGNMENT: First-come, first-served; group site by reservation

REGISTRATION: On-site self-registration or online (group site)

AMENITIES: Vault toilets, paved boat launch

PARKING: At campsites or group lots

FEES: $15/night (single), $60/night (group)

WHEELCHAIR ACCESS: Accessible restrooms

ELEVATION: 4,021'

RESTRICTIONS:

PETS: On leash only

FIRES: In rings only

ALCOHOL: Permitted

VEHICLES: Up to 34 feet

OTHER: 14-day stay limit; maximum 10 people, 2 vehicles/site (single) or 40 people, 10 vehicles/site (group); wood gathering prohibited

Delicate Arch is the flagship of Arches and, in more recent years, the poster child for Utah tourism. Its likeness can be seen on local business logos, bumper stickers, and even on Utah license plates. This 45-foot wide, 64-foot high sandstone arch sits on the rim of a large and steep-sided bowl. Ribbons of orange, tan, and buff run horizontally across the legs of the arch, adding details and highlights to the structure that keep you examining the formation over and over again. It's easy to see why many consider this one feature the single most-photographed item in Utah.

To reach Delicate Arch, enter the park from the turnoff just north of Moab on US 191 and take the paved road 11 miles to the junction for Wolfe Ranch and Delicate Arch. Turn right on this road and continue about a mile to the Wolfe Ranch parking area. Park and hike the 1.5 miles over steep, slick rock to Delicate Arch for an up-close-and-personal view. Bring plenty of water, and avoid going in the heat of the day as there's scarcely any shade. Better yet, go in the evening and see the arch at sunset.

If you can't make the 3-mile round-trip, just continue on the paved road past Wolfe Ranch for less than a mile to the Delicate Arch Viewpoint parking area. Here you can find more information at an interpretive display and enjoy the view of the arch from a distance. Or opt for a 1.5-mile round-trip hike to see the arch from a different vantage point.

Fiery Furnace is another popular hike in the park. This area showcases the "fins" of sandstone canyons—long rock peninsulas that tower above the canyon floor and drop off dramatically on each side. Park rangers offer guided walks of Fiery Furnace and recommend that no one enter on their own. Many hikers have become lost in the labyrinth of narrow trails. Those who do enter on their own must obtain a permit from park officials. To access Fiery Furnace, go back to the main park road and continue about 2.5 miles deeper into the park to the turnoff for Fiery Furnace. Talk to park officials at the visitor's center located at the park entrance to find out when guided tours of Fiery Furnace depart each day.

With landmark names like "Park Avenue," "Balanced Rock," "Devil's Garden," and "Dark Angel," you could spend days pursuing new adventures in Arches. Just be mindful of park rules. The actions of a few daredevils and attention-hungry individuals have resulted in the loss of life and caused the park service to tighten regulations; most notably, they have reemphasized that visitors are strictly prohibited from climbing on any named arch inside the park. Please obey the rules and take home photographs instead of fines—they make better souvenirs.

At the end of the day, when most park visitors are jamming into the park's Devil's Garden Campground, you can make your way back to Hittle Bottom and rest quietly for the night. With such a small number of sites, it will be a welcome refuge from the buzzing hoards of tourists back in town. You'll enjoy special seclusion by avoiding sites 2–4, which are right next to each other. Site 5 is tucked back beneath a tall cottonwood and surrounded by tamarisks, and site 10 is all by itself at the end of the campground loop.

If you don't want all the commotion of a national park, you can lounge around camp and enjoy the view of Fisher Towers, or you can put in your raft or kayak on the site's paved boat ramp. If you do enter the water, make sure that you know what's downstream: the Colorado River may look calm, but its swift-moving waters can be dangerous, especially during spring runoff.

Arches National Park: Hittle Bottom Campground

GETTING THERE

From I-70/US 6, take Exit 182 in Crescent Junction and drive south 29 miles on US 191. In Moab, just after you cross the Colorado River, turn left on UT 128 and drive east 23 miles to the campground entrance, on your left.

GPS COORDINATES: N38° 45.549' W109° 19.441'

Bowery Creek Campground

Beauty: ★★★★ / Privacy: ★★★★ / Quiet: ★★★ / Spaciousness: ★★★ / Security: ★★★ / Cleanliness: ★★★★

Baptize your outdoors-averse family members into the wonderful world of tall trees and open air.

As summertime brings high temperatures, Utahns head for higher elevations. For years, outdoors enthusiasts and heat refugees alike have been coming to Fish Lake for its crisp air and chilly waters. There are 40 campsites at Bowery Creek that welcome them each season with simple accommodations and a perfect location just minutes from the lake's shore.

There's no easy way to describe the configuration of this campground. Two access points lie along the main road, which arcs into a diamondlike loop and sprouts a triangle zigzag with a baby pyramid at one end and a circle at the other—the classic arched-diamond-ziggy triangasphere. At any rate, the layout makes its way up a hillside away from the lake and road, with a few choice views of the lake valley from scattered breaks in the aspen cover.

If views are your thing, try to snatch up site 41 or 42. These two sites, along with 22 others at Bowery Creek, are offered on a first-come, first-served basis. You'd better be one of the first to arrive, because this campground will fill up every weekend all summer long. Sites 32 and 33 are designated for tenters only, and while they're OK options, you'll probably find

Young aspens provide a feast for the eyes while the grill cooks up a feast of another kind.

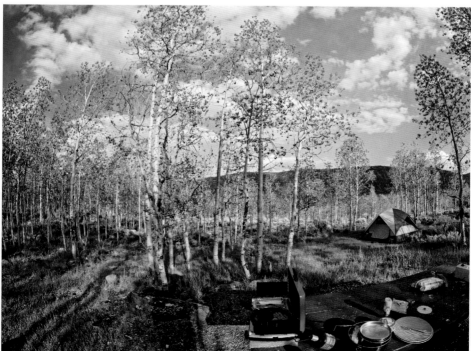

Photo: rovingmagpie/Flickr

KEY INFORMATION

LOCATION: FR 067, Loa, UT 84747

CONTACTS: 435-836-2800, tinyurl.com
/fishlakenfcamping; reservations: 877-444-
6777, recreation.gov

OPERATED BY: High Country Recreation for
Fishlake National Forest, Fremont River
Ranger District

OPEN: May–September

SITES: 40 (including 3 doubles and 3 triples)

EACH SITE: Picnic table, fire ring,
barbecue grill

ASSIGNMENT: First-come, first-served;
16 sites by reservation

REGISTRATION: On-site self-registration
or online

AMENITIES: Flush toilets, drinking water

PARKING: At campsites only

FEES: $15/night (single), $30/night (double),
$42/night (triple), $7.50/additional vehicle

WHEELCHAIR ACCESS: Sites 5 and 6,
restrooms

ELEVATION: 8,892'

RESTRICTIONS:

PETS: On leash only

FIRES: In fire rings only

ALCOHOL: Permitted

VEHICLES: Up to 150 feet

OTHER: 10-day stay limit; maximum
10 people/site (single), 20 people/site
(double), or 30 people/site (triple);
off-road vehicles prohibited

a more comfy spot elsewhere on the triangasphere—that is, if you don't mind the possibility of spending the night next to a Winnebago. Many of the sites are suited to RVs, but tents can occupy them as well. For campers with special-access needs, sites 5 and 6 have been made fully accessible.

Reservations are accepted for 10 single sites, 3 doubles, and 3 triples. Consider booking one of the larger camps for an extended camping trip or family affair. This is a great place to baptize your outdoors-averse family members into the wonderful world of tall trees and open air. There are modern restrooms at camp and convenience-store concessions available at the nearby Fish Lake Lodge.

The sky's the limit around Fish Lake. There are as many things to do there as there are days of the summer. The most obvious attraction is to grab your fishing rod and help the lake live up to its name. Fishing is a big draw here, both in summer when the campgrounds are full, and in winter when they're all closed up. The lake is Utah's biggest natural mountain lake, so it grows some good-sized lake trout. You could dedicate a lifetime to trying to figure out how to land these big boys, but ask around at the local lodge or tackle shop, or spend some time digging around online to shave a few years off of the endeavor. Lake trout have company; browns, rainbows, splake, and perch also swim these waters.

Not enough big fish? Johnson Valley Reservoir, just a few miles northeast of Fish Lake along UT 25, is planted with tiger muskie, a sterile hybrid of muskellunge and northern pike. These toothy critters are lean, mean eating machines. Currently, you can't even keep a tiger muskie at Johnson Valley unless it's more than 40 inches long.

Bring your mountain bike on this camp and choose from several popular trails. If you've got the time, the Mytoge Mountain Trail will take you on a 25-mile loop around the entire lake. It's no pedal in the park, though: a few climbs will have you digging deep, and a steep downhill section requires some delicate maneuvering. Give yourself 4 or 5 hours, depending on your fitness level. Bring lots of water or, even better, pack a lunch. Find the trailhead at Fish Lake Lodge.

Fishlake National Forest is peppered with little lakes and high mountain streams that receive only light-to-moderate recreational use. Forest Road 640 (Gooseberry Fremont Road) wanders through some of this territory, eventually passing Gooseberry Campground and connecting with I-70. Gooseberry Campground (not to be confused with Gooseberry Reservoir Campground, both in Manti–La Sal National Forest), is the busiest spot on this road and looks like a summer camp with its bunkhouses, meeting hall, restrooms, and picnic area. But side roads like Forest Road 040 to Rex Reservoir, Forest Road 350 to Lost Creek Reservoir, or the trails leaving from Gooseberry will give you more than enough hiking and sightseeing options.

The resort atmosphere at Fish Lake makes it hard to feel like you're really roughing it, but once you've ducked back into the campground, climbed into your tent, and pulled your sleeping bag tight up to your chin, you forget all that and just listen to the sounds of nature as they lull you to sleep.

Bowery Creek Campground

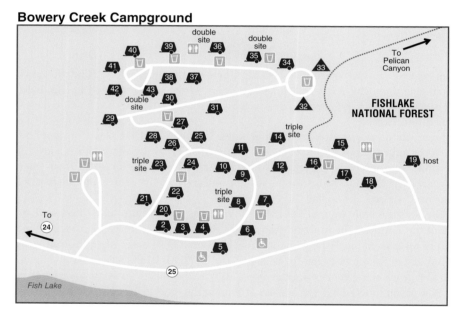

GETTING THERE

From the junction of UT 72 and UT 24 in Loa, head west 12.5 miles on UT 24. At the junction of UT 24 and UT 25, bear right (northeast) at the fork onto UT 25 and drive 9.6 miles to the campground, on your left. Two access points lie 0.3 mile apart on UT 25.

GPS COORDINATES: N38° 33.740′ W111° 42.426′

33

Bryce Canyon National Park:
PINE LAKE CAMPGROUND

Beauty: ★★★★ / Privacy: ★★★ / Quiet: ★★★★ / Spaciousness: ★★★★ / Security: ★★★★ / Cleanliness: ★★★★

This high-mountain campground is the perfect place to make your home base.

Pine Lake is a day-tripper's dream. It's located within a few hours' radius of two national parks, three state parks, and two national monuments, so time is the only restraint on how much exploring you can do. This high-mountain campground is the perfect place to make your home base and maximize your time in what is arguably Utah's most sensational outdoors corridor.

Pine Lake Campground isn't located in Bryce Canyon proper, but that's a positive. Both campgrounds in the park are actually quite nice, with new restrooms and are within walking distance to incredible hikes and vistas. But in summer the crowds there are swarming.

Aptly named for its location among spruce and towering ponderosa pine trees, Pine Lake is a cool and out-of-the-way spot in an otherwise hot and busy region of southern Utah. Most of the spots here are shaded and have good access to drinking water—a rarity among the region's more out-of-the-way campgrounds. At more than 8,100 feet in elevation, Pine Lake's nights will be brisk but a welcome change to warmer days. The only downside is that the campground doesn't typically open until Memorial Day or later, depending on the weather.

Pine Lake Campground has an upper and lower loop that piggyback one on top of the other. Sites 6–14 and 28–33 are located on the lower loop, 15–27 on the upper. Most of the individual sites here, along with the group sites, can be reserved ahead of time. The campground fills up on weekends, so make your reservations well in advance to ensure that you've got a place to stay. If not, dispersed camping is allowed beyond the lake, but sites are harder to find and more frequently buzzed by off-road vehicles along the Great Western Trail.

These rock spires call to mind upside-down icicles, or perhaps something out of Frank Herbert's *Dune*.

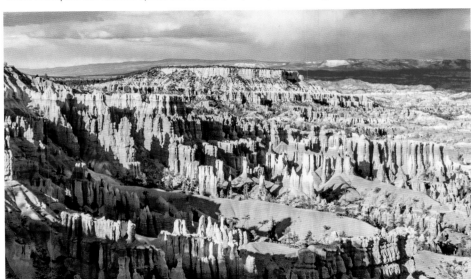

KEY INFORMATION

LOCATION: Just off Pine Lake Road (FR 132), Antimony, UT 84712

CONTACTS: 435-826-5400, tinyurl.com /dixienfcamp; reservations: 877-444-6777, recreation.gov

OPERATED BY: Scenic Canyons Recreation Service for Dixie National Forest, Escalante Ranger District

OPEN: Late May–October (depending on weather)

SITES: 28, plus 4 group sites and day-use area

EACH SITE: Picnic table, fire ring

ASSIGNMENT: First-come, first-served or by reservation

REGISTRATION: On-site self-registration or online

AMENITIES: Vault toilets, drinking water Memorial Day–Labor Day, primitive boat launch, group picnic/day-use area

PARKING: At campsites only

FEES: $15/night (single), $45/night (Clay Creek, Wild Iris, and Yellow Pine Group Sites), $90/night (Johns Valley Group Site), $5/additional vehicle; $2 day-use fee

WHEELCHAIR ACCESS: Not designated

ELEVATION: 8,150'

RESTRICTIONS:

PETS: On leash only

FIRES: In rings only

ALCOHOL: Permitted

VEHICLES: Up to 35 feet

OTHER: 14-day stay limit; maximum 8 people/ site (single), 50 people/site (Wild Iris and Yellow Pine Group Sites), or 100 people/site (Johns Valley Group Site); quiet hours 10 p.m.–6 a.m.

If you're staying during the week, try getting any site in the upper loop (except 22, which is right on the road). These are farthest away from the host, the lake, and other campers. If you'd rather get close to the water, try the lower loop. Sites 6–8 are the closest to the shore.

One of the best features of the campground is its proximity to Pine Lake. The shores of the lake are only a few minutes away—close enough to visit when you'd like, but far enough away that campers with little ones won't have to keep looking over their shoulder.

This pretty little lake is a great place to launch a canoe and get out on the open water. At 77 acres in surface area, it gives you plenty of space to paddle. Since powerboats of any kind are prohibited, paddle power rules the lake. Take along a fishing pole and try for one of the lake's resident rainbow or cutthroat trout. They can be a bit finicky but can usually be coaxed into playing tug-of-war when they get hungry at sunup and sundown.

Check current fishing regulations before wetting your line. Pine Lake has been the focus of some habitat restoration work in years past, and special regulations were placed to protect spawning trout, including the closure of the river that flows into the lake.

With each new day started at Pine Lake Campground, you have the best of southern Utah recreation at your fingertips. Most Pine Lake campers spend at least one day at Bryce Canyon National Park. The entrance to the park is just 17 miles away, back down UT 22. The National Park Service shuttle runs April–November, which means you'll drive just half an hour to the gates, park your car, and then take a bus into the park.

Bryce Canyon is truly a treat for the imagination. The exceptional geology of this area has earned it the honor of being one of Utah's most stellar places to snap a photo. Large spires defy gravity as they claw their way upward to the sky. The limestone rock has been so eroded that countless canyons, windows, and fins have been created here in the here in the Paunsaugunt Plateau. Jaw-dropping scenic turnouts and hikes with names like "Fairyland Loop" abound.

Other day trips might include Kodachrome Basin, Escalante Petrified Forest, or Anasazi State Park, to the east along UT 12. Grand Staircase–Escalante National Monument and Capitol Reef National Park are also located to the east on UT 12.

Consider driving UT 12 itself as a worthwhile day trip. This stretch of highway is often considered to be the most beautiful road in the United States as it wanders over narrow fins and narrowly carved rock face.

To the west, Red Canyon and Cedar Breaks National Monument are doable day trips. Both are postcard-worthy destinations that will have your camera finger clicking. Although a campground does exist at Red Canyon, you'll be glad you're up at Pine Lake when you see (and hear) the crowds that pass through the area immediately surrounding that area.

Plan your next family reunion at Pine Lake Campground, and you'll be the family hero. Four reservable group sites and a reservable day-use picnic area cater entirely to the needs of families, with large, open areas away from the waterfront and water spigots and restrooms nearby for convenience. Rather than have to sit around and listen all week long to stories about Aunt Margie's latest medical procedure, you can escape to a different adventure each day, or just head to the lake. The fresh air and comforting scenery should help you shake out images of Aunt Margie in a hospital gown.

Bryce Canyon National Park: Pine Lake Campground

GETTING THERE

From the intersection of Center Street and UT 12 (Main Street) in the town of Tropic, drive 7.5 miles northwest on UT 12. At the junction, turn right onto Johns Valley Road and drive 10.6 miles northeast on UT 22. Turn right at the brown campground sign onto Forest Road 132; in 5.4 miles, keep straight just past the intersection to reach the campground.

GPS COORDINATES: N37° 44.733' W111° 57.139'

34

Canyonlands National Park:
HAMBURGER ROCK CAMPGROUND

Beauty: ★★★★ / Privacy: ★★★★ / Quiet: ★★★ / Spaciousness: ★★★ / Security: ★★★★ /
Cleanliness: ★★★★★

Come on—how cool is it to say you've camped in a hamburger?

Hamburger Rock Campground is one of the most unusual campgrounds in Utah. Its name-sake: a squatty, circular stone that bears a resemblance to a giant burger with all the fixin's, inside the newly formed Bears Ears National Monument.

This burger's not just for looks; you can dive right into one of the Bureau of Land Management's seven campsites that are tucked into the nooks and crannies of the burger's perimeter, and you're perched near the boundary of Canyonlands National Park. Canyonlands is divided into three sections: Island in the Sky, which is the most popular and most visitor-friendly; The Needles, which has some measure of tourist attention; and The Maze, which is one of the most remote places in the entirety of the United States. Hamburger Rock is just 6 miles from the oft-overlooked Needles Visitor Center.

The tiny alcoves around the campground perimeter provide shelter from the sun and wind and keep you separated from other campers. In colder months, you may want to set up camp at either site 2 or site 3. You'll have the warm sunshine in camp for most of the day.

Where's the beef? It's right here at Hamburger Rock!

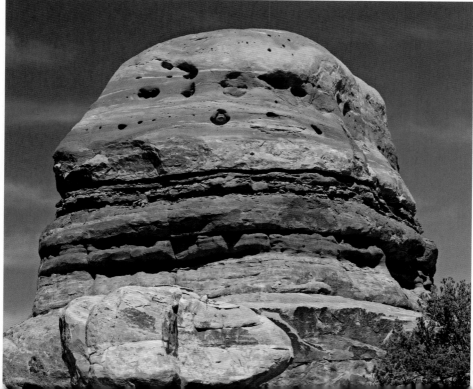

Photo: Wildnerdpix/Shutterstock

KEY INFORMATION

LOCATION: Lockhart Road north of UT 211, Monticello, UT 84535

OPERATED BY: Bureau of Land Management, Monticello Field Office

CONTACT: 435-587-1500, blm.gov/utah

OPEN: Year-round

SITES: 7

EACH SITE: Picnic table, fire ring

ASSIGNMENT: First-come, first-served; no reservations

REGISTRATION: On-site self-registration

AMENITIES: Pit toilets

PARKING: At campsites only

FEE: $10/night

WHEELCHAIR ACCESS: Not designated

ELEVATION: 4,866'

RESTRICTIONS:

PETS: On leash only

FIRES: In fire rings only

ALCOHOL: Permitted

VEHICLES: Up to 25 feet

OTHER: 14-day stay limit; maximum 6 people, 2 vehicles/site

The tradeoff is privacy, which dissipates in these two less-protected sites. Site 1 is definitely unique—if this giant sandstone rock is a hamburger, you'll be sleeping with the pickles and mayo! It's as if a small wedge has been nibbled away and site 1 tucks into the rounded rock formation. On the back side of the campground, sites 4 and 5 are also structured similarly, though to a lesser degree.

Amenities are basic here—a pit toilet on the east side of the campground and convenient road access set it apart from primitive dispersed camping in the region. That said, the toilet is tidy and quite a luxury where the vegetation is sparse. And come on—how cool is it to say you've camped in a hamburger?

Normally a bulgy little burger would look out of place, but Hamburger Rock fits in well in the Indian Creek area. Flat chocolate-chunk cliff walls, funky toadstool rock stands, and far-off mesas form a perfect backdrop. Be sure to check the latest land-management information as the future of Bears Ears has changed since it gained its much-deserved protection.

On one visit, I missed Hamburger Rock in the dark and rain and stayed dispersed-style in a cute little C-shaped alcove that I've affectionately nicknamed Fortune Cookie Campsite. While I had made the journey in the dark of night, I awoke the next morning to a cloudless sky and my first vision of the area by daylight. Breathtaking! Vibrant reds and oranges contrasted against the profoundly deep-blue sky, and I saw hundreds of tiny pools of water that filled the pockmarked sandstone surfaces surrounding me. This is the scenery of the Indian Creek area.

Plan on staying at Hamburger Rock for a while; there's plenty to explore. Most Hamburger Rockers do it by off-road vehicle, but you'll be better rewarded on foot. UT 211 hosts a bevy of trailheads, both marked and unmarked.

Follow UT 211 a few more miles and you'll enter the Needles District of Canyonlands National Park, where you'll find day hikes of all shapes and sizes, along with some of Utah's best backpacking possibilities. Your best bet is to find a good guidebook specific to the Canyonlands area and whittle down your choices. The Canyonlands website (nps.gov/cany) also has excellent downloadable overview maps in PDF format. Be vigilant in verifying park regulations regarding backcountry hiking and camping, because permits are required and, in some cases, must be reserved well in advance.

The drive to Hamburger Rock will test your tendency to stop and smell the roses. The sweetest rose along this journey is Newspaper Rock, which sits just off of UT 211, about 12.5 miles from the junction with US 163. This smooth, dark sandstone rock face is peppered with petroglyphs dating back some 2,000 years. They're not exclusive to one culture; Anasazi, Fremont, Navajo, and more-modern Anglo symbols are all represented in this hodge-podge of ancient writings. Whether it was an ancient newspaper or bulletin board or it held a more sacred role, no one knows for sure. Take a few minutes to gaze at the hundreds of petroglyphs on your way to the campground to make your own judgment.

Lockhart Road, the road to the campground, is easy to miss. It's an unassuming little turnoff marked only by a small informational kiosk a few hundred feet down the dirt road, directly off UT 211 on the right. The last time I was in the area, I managed to find the turnoff in the dark, although I passed right by the campground. Allow a few extra minutes just in case, pay attention, and you'll be just fine. For the GPS crowd, the turnoff is located at N38° 10.560' W109° 39.960'.

Canyonlands National Park: Hamburger Rock Campground

GETTING THERE

From the intersection of US 191 (Main Street) and US 491 (Center Street) in Monticello, go 14.5 miles north on US 191 and turn left onto UT 211. After about 29 miles, turn right onto Lockhart Road and drive 1.5 miles north to the campground entrance, on your right.

GPS COORDINATES: N38° 11.523' W109° 40.217'

35

⚐ Capitol Reef National Park:
FRUITA CAMPGROUND

Beauty: ★★★★ / Privacy: ★★ / Quiet: ★★ / Spaciousness: ★★ / Security: ★★★ / Cleanliness: ★★★★

Phenomenal scenery, fabulous hiking, and free fruit combine for a truly fantastic camping experience.

Fruita Campground in Capitol Reef National Park offers a one-of-a-kind camping experience. Where else can you view the marvels of a singular and gorgeous national park *and* wander through orchards eating ripe fruit to your belly's content?

As its name suggests, Fruita Campground sits among fruit—22 orchards spread over more than 60 acres that were first planted by Mormon pioneers as they settled the nearby community of Fruita in 1880. The National Park Service now maintains the approximately 2,700 trees as a Rural Historic Landscape, growing cherries, apricots, peaches, pears, apples, plums, mulberries, almonds, and walnuts.

The campground itself is in the heart of all the orchards and consists of three loops tucked between the Fremont River and road. Loops A and B sit right near the river and its footpath, while Loop C is separated from the river by the amphitheater.

Each campsite is a spur off of the paved loop road, with sites positioned one next to the other. A graveled parking space next to the lawn is where you'll set up your tent. You'll feel more like you're at a park than at a campground; this may be the most RV-friendly site in the book, and you'll be surrounded by tall trees and manicured grass. But to stay among the orchards, eat your fill of fruit, and soak in the charm of the Fremont River Valley is worth the tradeoff.

Stay at the campground, and you can take advantage of the park's official invitation, as found in one of the park's brochures: "You are welcome to stroll in any unlocked orchard and consume ripe fruit while in the orchards." Bring on the cherries! Bring on the apricots! Bring on the Pepto-Bismol!

Fruita Campground gives you plenty to see—and savor.

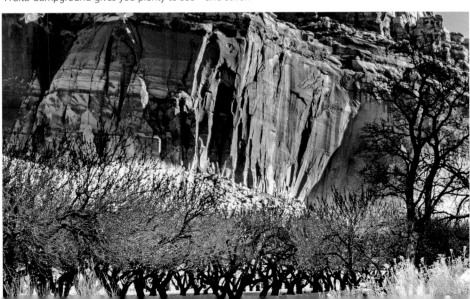

KEY INFORMATION

LOCATION: South of UT 24, Teasdale, UT 84773

CONTACTS: 435-425-3791, nps.gov/care; reservations: 877-444-6777, recreation.gov

OPERATED BY: Capitol Reef National Park, National Park Service

OPEN: Year-round

SITES: 71 (including 7 walk-ins), plus 1 group site

EACH SITE: Picnic table, fire ring (standard) or barbecue stand (walk-in)

ASSIGNMENT: First-come, first-served; group site by reservation

REGISTRATION: On-site self-registration or online (group site)

FACILITIES: Flush toilets, drinking water, visitor center, amphitheater, garbage service

PARKING: At campsites; overflow parking available

FEES: $20/night (single), $75/night minimum (group site)

WHEELCHAIR ACCESS: Sites 26 and 63, restrooms

ELEVATION: 5,400'

RESTRICTIONS:

PETS: On leash only

FIRES: In fire rings/grills only

ALCOHOL: Permitted

VEHICLES: Up to 52 feet

OTHER: 14-day stay limit in season, 30 additional days/year off-season; maximum 8 people/site (single) or 40 people/site (group); hammocks may be hung during daylight hours only

If you'd like to take home some genuine Capitol Reef fruit for friends and neighbors, there are self pick-and-pay stations for any fruit you take home. Some visitors plan their trips around the harvest time of their favorite fruit. Although the weather can change availability, the schedule below shows the approximate flowering and harvest dates of different fruits. For the latest information, call the park at 435-425-3791 and press *1*, then *5* in order to reach the recorded fruit hotline.

FRUIT	FLOWERING	HARVEST	FRUIT	FLOWERING	HARVEST
Cherries	3/31–4/19	6/11–7/7	Pears	3/31–5/3	8/7–9/8
Apricots	2/27–3/20 (early) 3/7–4/13 (regular)	6/27–7/22 (early) 6/28–7/18 (regular)	Apples	4/10–5/6	9/4–10/17
Peaches	3/26–4/23	8/4–9/6			

Each of the 71 individual sites is available on a first-come, first-served basis; the group site can be reserved online and holds up to 40 people. Around the time when the first edition of this book was published, Capitol Reef was "discovered," and visitorship has gone from under a half million to almost one million people per year. Do yourself a favor: take that extra day off work and get into Fruita by Thursday morning. You'll avoid the risk of finding the campground full and you'll have an extra-long weekend to enjoy the area.

Capitol Reef National Park is most famous for the 100-mile wrinkle in the earth's surface that it sits on, known as Waterpocket Fold. This "kink" in the earth's crust, created by the same force that lifted the Colorado Plateau, is home to brightly colored cliffs, rock spires, domes, arches, and monoliths that defy the imagination.

Hikers enjoy a multitude of opportunities and some of the finest desert hiking available in the state. Cathedral Valley, in the northern part of the park, is accessible only by dirt road—from the west over Thousand Lake Mountain (see Elkhorn Campground, page 129) or from the east on rocky roads that ford various rivers. Massive monoliths define this region of Capitol Reef. Muley Twist Canyon, a popular attraction in the south of the park, is a challenging desert hike that will have you discovering exciting arches and new views around every turn.

Camping in the backcountry is allowed, but you must first obtain a free permit from park officials. Be prepared for rough conditions on any hike or backcountry adventure. Water is scarce in many parts of the park, so bring plenty of your own.

If you'd rather not take on the trails of Capitol Reef, there's plenty to do around Fruita Campground. Take the 25-mile round-trip scenic drive to view Waterpocket Fold from the comfort of your own car. This 2-hour outing leaves from the campground and puts you into some inspiring landscape. Be sure to get the printed drive guide from the visitor center before you go.

Near the campground, some of the original structures built by early settlers have been restored and are open to view. Peek in at the old Fruita Schoolhouse and blacksmith shop, stop by the Ripple Rock Nature Center, and be sure grab a freshly baked mini–fruit pie at the Gifford Homestead. Many cultural presentations, children's activities, and handmade sales items are offered each day. Check with the visitor center for a detailed schedule.

Few places illustrate the diversity of Utah's camping opportunities better than Fruita, where phenomenal scenery, fabulous hiking, and free fruit combine for a truly fantastic camping experience.

Capitol Reef National Park: Fruita Campground

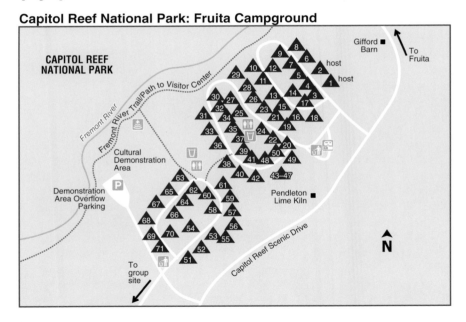

GETTING THERE

From the intersection of UT 12 and UT 24 in Torrey, drive 9.8 miles east on UT 24 to the entrance of Capitol Reef National Park. Turn right and drive 1.5 miles south past the visitor center to the campground, on your right.

GPS COORDINATES: N38° 16.973' W111° 14.915'

36

Cedar Canyon Campground

Beauty: ★★★★ / Privacy: ★★★ / Quiet: ★★★ / Spaciousness: ★★★★ / Security: ★★★ / Cleanliness: ★★★★

Cedar Canyon is best enjoyed from the comfort of a camp chair while sitting around the fire.

Cedar Canyon Campground is the epitome of off-the-highway family camping. Located just 13 miles from nearby Cedar City, it's a special little place by the side of the road that allows young and old campers alike to reconnect with nature.

Set amid spruce, fir, and aspen trees, some of the campsites here get plenty of shade and block out views of the traffic on nearby UT 14. Crow Creek lies between the campsites and the highway as well. Its delightful little song also mutes out the sounds of cars as well as other campers.

The Pink Cliffs of Cedar Breaks National Monument

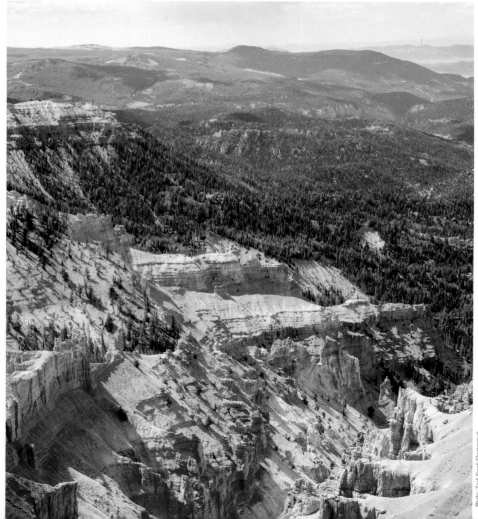

Photo: Zack Frank/Shutterstock

KEY INFORMATION

LOCATION: UT 14, Cedar City, UT 84720

CONTACTS: 435-865-3200, tinyurl.com
/dixienfcamp; reservations: 877-444-6777,
recreation.gov

OPERATED BY: Scenic Canyons Recreation
Service for Dixie National Forest, Cedar City
Ranger District

OPEN: Late May–October (depending
on weather)

SITES: 17 (including 5 doubles), plus
1 group site

EACH SITE: Picnic table, fire ring

ASSIGNMENT: First-come, first-served or
by reservation

REGISTRATION: On-site self-registration
or online

AMENITIES: Vault toilets, drinking water
Memorial Day–Labor Day, garbage service

PARKING: At campsites only

FEES: $17/night (single), $34/night (double),
$55/night (group)

WHEELCHAIR ACCESS: Restrooms only

ELEVATION: 7,940'

RESTRICTIONS:

PETS: On leash only

FIRES: In fire rings only

ALCOHOL: Permitted

VEHICLES: Up to 40 feet

OTHER: 14-day stay limit; maximum 8 people/
site (single), 16 people/site (double), or
35 people/site (group); off-road vehicles
must be trailered in and out

Crow Creek is not a fishable stream, but anglers need not despair. Just a few miles far-ther up the highway are many different fishing opportunities. At only 11 miles away, Navajo Lake is a fun day trip. There are campgrounds closer to this skinny lake, but they tend to be a bit more raucous than Cedar Canyon. Navajo Lake yields high-quality rainbow, brook, and splake trout (a hybrid of brook and lake trout) but can also be prone to problems in drought years. With a few good water years, however, this oft-overlooked fishing hole churns out some big brutes.

Fishing isn't really the main draw at Cedar Canyon; it's the good old-fashioned camp-ing that brings people up UT 14. The sites are spurred along a paved road. About a quar-ter of the 19 sites are to the left of the entrance road, the rest to the right. The sites could be better masked from each other, but they provide plenty of space to spread your gear, stretch out, and relax.

There are sites to accommodate most family or group sizes here; just be sure to pay attention when picking your site. Sites 5, 9, 12, 15, and 18 are doubles, and 19 is a group site that holds 35 people. All sites can be reserved ahead of time, or you can show up and hope for empty spots on a first-come, first-served basis.

The campsites here are worn in but not worn down; to the contrary, the campground is tidy and well maintained. The drinking water is fresh—piped in from a nearby spring—and the toilets are shipshape. There are enough open areas here that kids or anxious adults can spread out and explore. With its location, pleated up against the hill behind it, and a healthy mix of open air and wooded space, Cedar Canyon could host a killer game of steal the flag.

While you're staying at Cedar Canyon, take the opportunity to visit nearby Cedar Breaks National Monument. Go east on UT 14 about 5 miles and turn left at the junction with UT 148. The monument entrance is 4 miles north on UT 148.

Cedar Breaks is simply stunning. Here, you'll see a gargantuan amphitheater carved from the eroded Pink Cliffs of the Claron Formation. At its high point, the rim of the massive valley sits at 10,000 feet above sea level, but the canyon plunges 2,000 feet before your eyes. Note the dramatic contrast between the pinkish layered canyon walls and the dark-green Engelmann spruces and subalpine firs that dot the rim and tumbling landscape before you.

Visit Cedar Breaks in early July, and you'll also see great colors of blossoming wildflowers in the meadows. Among the most common are bright-yellow sunflowers and potentilla, blue lupines and bluebells, and purple larkspur, although the time and focus of your visit will dictate what colors you see.

Cedar Canyon Campground is near the Virgin River Rim Trail, a 32.5-mile trail that parallels UT 14 and is quite popular with mountain bikers. Doing the whole trail by bike in one day is probably too ambitious, but sections can be done as an out-and-back. Start from either the Woods Ranch Recreation Area, a few miles below the campground, or the Strawberry Point Trailhead, 9 miles up Forest Service Road 60 (Strawberry Road), about 20 miles farther up UT 14. This trail is one of Dixie National Forest's best-kept secrets for exceptional canyon hiking and photography.

While it's surrounded by all kinds of adventure, Cedar Canyon is best enjoyed from the comfort of a camp chair while sitting around the fire, marshmallow roaster in hand. The soothing river and crisp mountain air can lull even the most hardcore thrill-seeker into a roasted marshmallow–induced sleep.

Cedar Canyon Campground

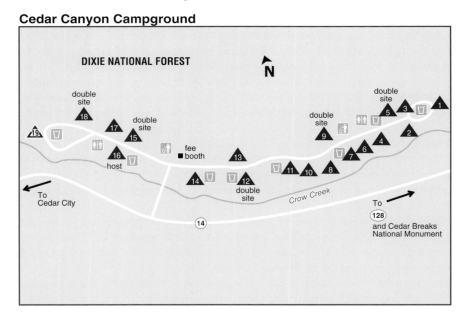

GETTING THERE

From the intersection of UT 130 (Main Street) and UT 14 (East Center Street) in Cedar City, a couple of blocks east of the Southern Utah University campus, drive 12.2 miles east on UT 14 to the campground entrance, on your left.

GPS COORDINATES: N37° 35.485′ W112° 54.259′

37

Cowboy Camp Campground

Beauty: ★★★★★ / Privacy: ★★★ / Quiet: ★★★★ / Spaciousness: ★★ / Security: ★★★ / Cleanliness: ★★★★

If these hills could talk, they'd tell you about all the cowboys they'd seen.

In days of the Wild West, very few places were as wild as this part of Utah. Indeed, if these hills could talk, they'd tell you about all the cowboys they'd seen over the years, riding over the rough desert terrain. Today, you can camp on that same soil once ridden by some of the most storied figures of the 19th century.

Cowboy Camp is a simple but sweet little seven-site campground just off UT 313, some 20 miles from US 191. If you've never taken the drive up UT 313, it's worth it even if you plan to camp elsewhere. The road climbs from the valley floor and winds around hairpin turns where it's been carved into the red-and-orange rock walls. As you make your way to the campground, you rise more than 1,500 feet and are rewarded with stellar views, along with plenty of scenic turnouts to take advantage.

The first time I stayed here, I arrived well after dark and nearly missed the turnoff. It's poorly marked (just a small brown sign reading NO TRAILERS with a campground symbol), and once you turn, you're warned of a rough road not suitable for trailers. I quickly set up my tent and went to sleep. When I awoke, I was greeted with some jaw-dropping views of the desert to the west. The campground is perched on the ledge of a massive shelf and looks out over a flat landscape, with gnarled rock formations in the distance. With those precious golden hues found only at dawn, I just stood and stared at the view.

Cowboy Camp combines modest amenities with extravagant scenic beauty.

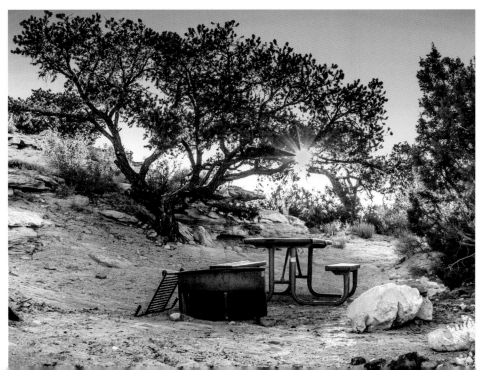

KEY INFORMATION

LOCATION: Just off UT 313, Moab, UT 84532

CONTACT: 435-259-2100, blm.gov/utah

OPERATED BY: Bureau of Land Management, Moab Field Office

OPEN: Year-round

SITES: 7

EACH SITE: Picnic table, fire ring

ASSIGNMENT: First-come, first-served; no reservations

REGISTRATION: On-site self-registration

FACILITIES: Pit toilets

PARKING: At campsites only

FEE: $15/night

WHEELCHAIR ACCESS: Accessible restroom

ELEVATION: 6,129'

RESTRICTIONS:

PETS: On leash only

FIRES: In fire rings only

ALCOHOL: Permitted

VEHICLES: No RVs or trailers

OTHER: 14-day stay limit; maximum 10 people, 2 vehicles/site

You'll pass other camping opportunities along the way, with several others in the vicinity. Horsethief Campground was included in the first edition of this book, but it has since been "discovered," so to speak, and can be full of bigger vehicles and more people. You'll appreciate the solitude of Cowboy in contrast; most of the sites are spaced far from each other. If solitude is what you're after, site 7 is the one you seek. It's at the very end of the short campground road and sits off by itself. Site 1 will also provide plenty of space from your neighbors, but it's relatively close to the highway and you'll hear the cars passing by. Each site is equipped with a fire ring, a picnic table, and space to spread out. There are pit toilets but no water.

Cowboy Camp may not have much in the way of amenities, but its location is second to none. It's an easy day trip from here to Dead Horse Point State Park and both Canyonlands and Arches National Parks. Canyonlands consists of three districts: Island in the Sky, The Needles, and The Maze. You'll be a few miles outside of Island in the Sky, which is the most car-friendly and civilized sector. Drive the scenic road, or park and take the hike to Mesa Arch, especially at sunrise. You won't be alone, but considering the scenery, you'll hardly have to wonder why. Bring your camera to snap some shots of Shafer Canyon, Green River, and Grand View Point Overlooks. Although cameras can't do justice to the buttes, bluffs, and beautiful canyons, your friends will still have fits of jealousy when you show them your snapshots.

Take the time to head into Dead Horse Point State Park, too. Here, you'll be reminded that it's not necessarily heights you're afraid of but looking down to great depths. You'll enjoy awesome views from the edge of a cliff that plunges 2,000 feet to the Colorado River below. According to one legend, horses came to this point and were so thirsty they jumped off the high plateau to reach the water below, hence the park's grisly name. Views are especially breathtaking at sunrise and sunset, when the light creeps up and down the jagged canyon walls, igniting them in brilliant hues of orange and red before leaving them in a stately silhouette against the night sky. Check the information board at the visitor center, where the staff updates the sunset and sunrise times daily.

Once you've seen the more established sites, you can still use this campground as a base to explore the lesser-known parts of the area. The landscape around Moab is packed with winding trails that beg to be explored by four-wheel-drive or mountain bike, or on foot.

The horses of yesteryear have been traded for more horsepower today, but you could pick a different road spur nearly every day and never run out of things to explore in this vast and varied part of planet Earth.

The old horse thieves and outlaws are all ghosts. Those dusty trails are two-lane highways. But with a can of beans, a harmonica, and the near-infinite views of the American West at your campsite, you might just come home a little bit cowboy.

Cowboy Camp Campground

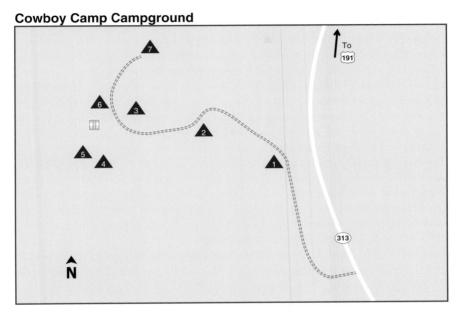

GETTING THERE

From I-70/US 6, take Exit 182 in Crescent Junction and drive south 20 miles on US 191. Turn right (west) and take UT 313 for 14 miles; then turn right into the campground.

GPS COORDINATES: N38° 33.636' W109° 47.616'

38

⚠ Dalton Springs Campground

Beauty: ★★★★ / Privacy: ★★★ / Quiet: ★★★ / Spaciousness: ★★★ / Security: ★★★★ / Cleanliness: ★★★★

The Abajo Mountains are the first mountains to become snow-free after winter.

There's a lot to be said for being first, and the Abajo Mountains (sometimes also called the Blue Mountains) have their own first to claim: they're the first mountains in Utah to become snow-free after winter. While the rest of the state languishes under snowpack, Dalton Springs Campground quietly sheds its snow and typically offers some of the first high-mountain experiences for campers and hikers who've been itching with spring fever.

Located just west of the city of Monticello (less than 50 air miles from the border of Arizona) at an altitude of 8,400 feet, this small campground can open as early as the first week of May, according to 35 years of snowpack data. Compare that with late June or July for the alpine campgrounds in the northern part of the state, and you have a perfect destination for a spring when you've just been pining for a campground with pines.

The campground itself is set up as a loop inside of a loop off of Forest Road 105. Shaded by pines, oak, and aspen, there are 14 regular campsites and 2 double sites (1 and 14). Sites 4–13 are located on an inner loop, with numbers 5, 7, 8, and 11 offering pull-through convenience. Stay in site 9, 10, or 12, and you'll be a bit removed from the camp by backing up toward the mountain. Sites 15 and 16 are also nice, though somewhat less private; plus, you'll have to walk farther to get water from site 16.

There's plenty to do in the Abajo Mountains. Just up the road past Buckboard Campground (a viable option if Dalton Springs is full) are Monticello and Foy Lakes. Both are

Glen Canyon National Recreation Area viewed from Dalton Springs

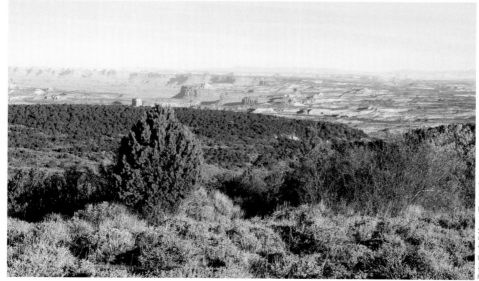

Photo: Claudio Del Luongo/Shutterstock

KEY INFORMATION

LOCATION: Just south of FR 101, Monticello, UT 84535

CONTACT: 435-587-2041, tinyurl.com/mantilasalcamping

OPERATED BY: Manti–La Sal National Forest, Monticello Ranger District

OPEN: May–October (water availability varies)

SITES: 16 (including 2 doubles)

EACH SITE: Picnic table, metal fire ring

ASSIGNMENT: First-come, first-served; no reservations

REGISTRATION: On-site self-registration

AMENITIES: Vault toilets, water, garbage service

PARKING: At campsites only

FEE: $10/night (single), $12/night (double)

WHEELCHAIR ACCESS: Not designated

ELEVATION: 8,402'

RESTRICTIONS:

PETS: On leash only

FIRES: In fire rings only

ALCOHOL: Permitted

VEHICLES: No restrictions

OTHER: 14-day stay limit; no saddle or pack animals

---

quite small but offer fun fishing for planted rainbow trout. Monticello Lake is just off the road. Foy is straight past the fork. The unobstructed views at Foy Lake, which is located at the crest of a hill, are especially noteworthy because of the lake. Look off into the distance and watch the mountains tumble down to the valley and turn shades of amber and red.

Drive around to the south side of the mountain toward Nizhoni Campground, and you'll find the larger Recapture Reservoir and the nearby Red Cliffs and Anasazi ruins. You could just as easily spend the day hiking amongst the mountain pines, as you could driving down the mountain and popping into a national park or monument.

Make sure to get up early in the morning before sunrise and take the drive toward Canyonlands National Park. Turn left out of the campground and drive west past Monticello Lake. After turning right at the fork, you'll begin your descent off the mountain. After only a few miles, you'll round bends in the road with astonishing views of the Needles District of Canyonlands. Layered red-rock canyons, each more distant than the last, weave together to create a dramatic sandstone skyline. At sunrise, watch the top of each of these layered canyons come to life with light and then slowly become illuminated down to their base. Pull over at any of the graded turnouts to take it all in. Come prepared with extra batteries for your camera—you may need them.

There are opportunities to hike in the Abajo Mountains, but you'll have to search to find them. Though more typically known for its horse trails, this area can offer some surprises for hikers who are willing to work. For an easy-to-find trail that takes you to the 11,362-foot Abajo Peak, turn left out of the campground and go about a half mile to Forest Road 079, also known as North Canyon Road; it's on the left side of the road. Park here and begin your ascent toward the peak. After about 3 miles, you can leave the road on a faint footpath, or continue on the more established route. Once you summit, you'll enjoy views of the mountains and surrounding colorful canyons.

Dalton Springs is a practical alternative if you're visiting Canyonlands. Campgrounds near the park are scorching-hot in the summer, and the Abajos provide a welcome respite from the sun. If you don't mind a beautiful 45-minute drive to the Needles District that meanders through juniper and then aspens and pines, stay above the heat and chaos by choosing Dalton Springs as your base camp.

Dalton Springs Campground

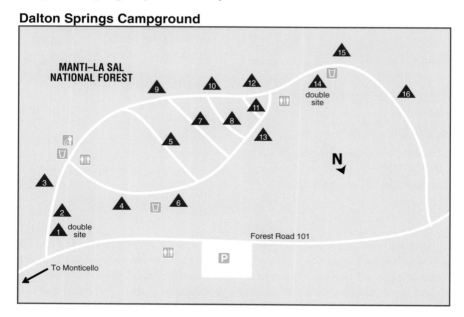

GETTING THERE

From I-70/US 6, take Exit 182 in Crescent Junction and drive south 86 miles on US 191. In Monticello, just after the brown MOUNTAIN RECREATION/CANYONLANDS NATIONAL PARK sign, turn right on West 200 South (FR 101) and drive 6 miles west on a paved road to the campground.

GPS COORDINATES: N37° 52.435' W109° 25.976'

39

⛺ Elkhorn Campground

Beauty: ★★★★★ / Privacy: ★★★ / Quiet: ★★★★ / Spaciousness: ★★★ / Security: ★★★★★ /
Cleanliness: ★★★★

Solitude is the main attraction at Elkhorn, and Thousand Lake Mountain offers it in spades.

No one visits Elkhorn by accident. The dirt road to the campground is accessed from a sel-dom-used stretch of highway and winds continually as it climbs 9 intimidating miles through the trees and passes by deep blue ponds characteristic of the rarely discussed Thousand Lake Mountain. It's remote and it's isolated. In other words, it's almost perfect.

Elkhorn is the only established campground on Thousand Lake. The campsites here sit at almost 10,000 feet in altitude in a needle-shaped configuration. Surprisingly, water is available at this campground from several spigots in the camp, and the restrooms have been redone to accommodate campers with disabilities.

The only thing that would make Elkhorn better would be spreading the sites out a little far-ther from each other. Still, being so high above and far away from civilization, you can hardly complain. Bring along your favorite novel—or sit at camp writing your own—and the only distraction you might have would be the overwhelming beauty of the forest around you. The campers and hunters who frequent the mountain also have a quiet respect for one another, so security isn't a big concern. Keep clear of the main road and OHVs won't be a bother, either.

Sites 5–7 serve up the best privacy at Elkhorn. They're sheltered from each other by big shady pines. If you've booked the group area (a steal at only $35), you can expect to be out in the open as it's met on its front side by a large meadow and the road to the nearby ranger field station.

Elkhorn Campground abuts the Monument Valley.

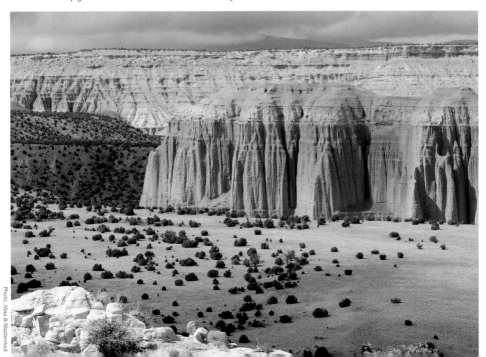

Photo: Nina B/Shutterstock

KEY INFORMATION

LOCATION: FR 210 just off of FR 206, Loa, UT 84747

CONTACTS: 435-836-2800, tinyurl.com /fishlakenfcamping; reservations: 877-444-6677, recreation.gov

OPERATED BY: Fishlake National Forest, Fremont River Ranger District

OPEN: Memorial Day–Labor Day

SITES: 7, plus 1 group site

EACH SITE: Picnic table, fire ring

ASSIGNMENT: First-come, first-served; group site by reservation

REGISTRATION: On-site self-registration or online (group site)

AMENITIES: Vault toilets, drinking water

PARKING: At campsites only

FEE: None for single sites, $35 minimum for group site

WHEELCHAIR ACCESS: Restrooms only

ELEVATION: 9,820'

RESTRICTIONS:

PETS: On leash only

FIRES: In fire rings only

ALCOHOL: Permitted

VEHICLES: Up to 70 feet

OTHER: 14-day stay limit; maximum 8 people/ site (single) or 75 people/site (group)

Solitude is the main attraction at Elkhorn, and Thousand Lake Mountain offers it in spades. Pick any trail or dirt road and follow it to your explorer heart's content. The only traffic you're bound to see involves people taking the scenic route over the mountain to Capitol Reef National Park's secluded Cathedral Valley. You'll have passed that turnoff on your way into Elkhorn, so unless you head back down the way you came, you can avoid this group completely.

Consider visiting Cathedral Valley while you're here, though. This awesome part of the national park is accessed on Forest Road 22 and boasts some mammoth-size monoliths made of Entrada sandstone that resemble every bit the impressive facades of the world's most ornate cathedrals. Elkhorn is a great place to stage your stay if you like a cooler place to spend your nights. You'll need a high-clearance four-wheel drive vehicle to visit the lonesome and harsh terrain of the sometimes-sandy, sometimes-muddy Cathedral Valley. If you don't have one, at least pull over to the side of the road at one of the many scenic turnoffs on Thousand Lake Mountain and take a picture.

On a particular visit in the early summer some years ago, I had to chuckle at the reservation notice posted on the group site; it was dated for September of the previous year. Apparently, Labor Day weekend was the last time anyone had been at the group area. On the off chance that you do find Elkhorn booked, there are almost infinite places to pull off for dispersed camping—sans the convenience of potties and water.

Near the campground is a small trail leading up the hill to Blue Lake. It's doable by four-wheel drive vehicle, but short enough to be refreshing on foot. It's about a mile-and-a-half hike to Blue, then another 1.5 to Neff Reservoir. You'll also see several small ponds along the way. Bring your fishing pole along and you'll be rewarded by hungry little brook trout. Other stocked lakes in the area include Blind Lake, Deep Creek Lake, Elkhorn Lake, Grass Lake, and Round Lake. Although Thousand Lake Mountain doesn't have as many lakes as Boulder Mountain to the south (in fact, some conjecture that the names of the two were transposed when recorded by early surveyors), there are still plenty of opportunities to test the waters for feisty fishies.

Bring along some bug spray, just to be sure. Nothing will ruin the peace and quiet of this special place faster than the constant buzz-land-slap routine that mosquitoes evoke. Also be sure to have a good rain jacket and some warmer clothes. You wouldn't think that in a place surrounded by hot and dusty desert you could get that cold, but at 10,000 feet, all bets are off.

Nineteenth-century English poet Christina Rossetti once wrote that "Silence is more musical than any song." While I don't think she ever visited Thousand Lake Mountain, I am certain that she would appreciate the symphony of silence available at the remote little Elkhorn Campground.

Elkhorn Campground

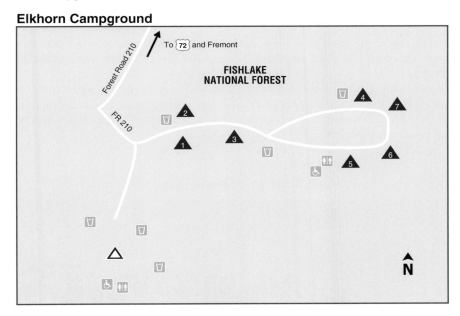

GETTING THERE

From the junction of UT 72 and UT 24 in Loa, take UT 72 northeast, passing through the town of Fremont. In 11.5 miles, turn right just after the brown campground sign onto Forest Road 206, heading east. In 3.1 miles, bear right (south) at the intersection to continue on FR 206; 1.8 miles farther, keep straight at a second intersection to continue south on this road. In 2.7 miles, bear right at a third intersection onto FR 210 to reach the campground.

GPS COORDINATES: N38° 27.822' W111° 27.425'

40

Goblin Valley State Park Campground

Beauty: ★★★★ / Privacy: ★ / Quiet: ★★★ / Spaciousness: ★★ / Security: ★★★ / Cleanliness: ★★★★★

Goblin Valley excites the mind and enlivens the imagination with images of oddly shaped desert hoodoos.

Imagine a place where little stone creatures dot the landscape like an eclectic mix of squatty snowmen, magical mushrooms, and tiny huts. Sounds pretty bizarre, right? I don't think they'll be putting "bizarre" in their brochure anytime soon, but that's definitely one way to describe Goblin Valley State Park.

These strange stone formations, commonly referred to as hoodoos, are actually made of eroded Entrada sandstone, worn from former highlands and deposited on the flat valley floor. The alternating layers of sandstone, siltstone, and shale now remain in the form of fantastic rock formations that seem to bubble up from the earth, like warts on the desert landscape.

The campground here in the valley of hoodoos is a top-notch facility, with a small visitor center, modern flush toilets and shower facilities, and a shade pavilion in each campsite. But while Goblin Valley is undoubtedly a comfortable place to camp, the downside is that heavy crowds makes camping cramped.

The hoodoos of Goblin Valley really do resemble otherworldly creatures.

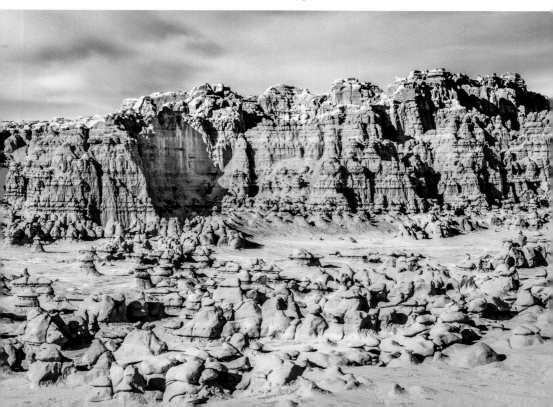

KEY INFORMATION

LOCATION: Goblin Valley Road, Green River, UT 84525-0637

CONTACTS: 435-275-4584, stateparks.utah .gov/parks/goblin-valley; reservations: 800-322-3770, reserveamerica.com

OPERATED BY: Goblin Valley State Park

OPEN: Year-round

SITES: 22, plus 2 yurts and 1 group site

EACH SITE: Picnic table, shade covering, fire ring

ASSIGNMENT: First-come, first-served or by reservation

REGISTRATION: On-site self-registration or online

AMENITIES: Visitor center, flush toilets, showers, drinking water

PARKING: At campsites only

FEE: $25/night (single), $85/night (group), $101/night (yurt), $15/additional vehicle

ELEVATION: 5,200'

WHEELCHAIR ACCESS: Site 22 and yurt 2, restrooms

RESTRICTIONS:

PETS: On leash only

FIRES: In fire rings only

ALCOHOL: Permitted

VEHICLES: Up to 50 feet

OTHER: 14-day stay limit; maximum 5 people/ site (yurt), 8 people/site (single), or 35 people/site (group)

The campground comprises a single loop with some sites spurred individually and others sharing a common parking area. It's clean and very well maintained, but the sites are squished together and privacy is lacking (hence one star in this category). If at all possible, try for site 12 or 19—the former allows you to tuck your tent behind a rock wall and shield yourself from your neighbors, and the latter sits all by itself at the last corner of the campground loop. The sites are also on the smallish side, though the shade pavilion and picnic table provide enough space for you to set out the essentials.

The vegetation around the campground is sparse, but it provides a good lesson in desert survival. The hardy plants that manage to eke out a life in the desert are well adapted to long dry spells and expend little energy to grow. Look around for Mormon tea (a type of ephedra— not the type used to make diet pills), Russian thistle, Indian ricegrass, and different species of cacti.

Spring and fall are the best times to visit Goblin Valley. Summers are swelteringly hot, with little reprieve from the blazing sun. Temperatures often reach the low 100s, although at night they can fall to the mid-60s. Winter would also make a unique visit, as it has been known to snow within the park. Seeing little goblins with puffy white hats would be worth the inconvenience of a little desert mud and frigid nighttime temperatures.

Reservations are accepted four months in advance and are strongly recommended—the park has been packed each time I've visited, whether weekend or weekday. Because of its remote location, there aren't any other established campgrounds with amenities in the area, although dispersed camping is always an option.

If you can adjust to constantly seeing and being seen by your camping neighbors, you'll fall in love with the geology of Goblin Valley. Drive to the observation point southeast of the campground, and you'll marvel at the hundreds of hoodoos below. An interpretive display explains in detail how the formations were created, and the wooden deck provides the perfect place to take pictures. Every so often, a tour bus drops off visitors who descend on the valley floor, so take advantage of the convenience of your camp and get the coveted people-less photo. When the sun has nearly set, you'll get eerie pictures of the ghostlike shadows cast by the odd sandstone ogres.

If you'd rather set out on foot, the park offers three trails: Carmel Canyon, a 1.5-mile loop from the parking area to the desert floor; Curtis Bench, an easy 2.1-mile out-and-back trail along the Curtis formation; and Entrada Canyon, a 1.3-mile trail to the goblins from the campground. Each one offers a different perspective on the distinctive rock structures.

Goblin Valley excites the mind and enlivens the imagination with images of oddly shaped desert hoodoos. They've been likened to mushrooms, warts, cottages, and chess pieces. What will you see on your visit?

Goblin Valley State Park Campground

GETTING THERE

From I-70, take Exit 149 just west of Green River (182 miles south of Salt Lake City), and drive southwest on UT 24. In 24.2 miles, turn right (west) onto Temple Mountain Road at the sign for Goblin Valley State Park. In 5.2 miles, turn left (south) onto Goblin Valley Road, and follow it 6.7 miles into Goblin Valley State Park. Then make a quick right to reach the campground, 0.2 mile ahead on your left.

GPS COORDINATES: N38° 34.336' W110° 42.740'

41

Lonesome Beaver Campground

Beauty: ★★★★ / Privacy: ★★★ / Quiet: ★★★★ / Spaciousness: ★★★ / Security: ★★★★ / Cleanliness: ★★★★★

However you enjoy Lonesome Beaver, you'll be one of the few who has.

Whimsical name aside, Lonesome Beaver is a bit of an oddity—but not in a bad way. Its location deep in southern Utah, coupled with the fact that it's a Bureau of Land Management (BLM) campground, would lead you to believe it's a dusty-desert locale full of sage, piñon pine, and plenty of hot temperatures. Au contraire: this small, secluded campground in the Henry Mountains is literally an oasis in southern Utah.

At more than 8,000 feet in elevation, Lonesome Beaver is smack-dab in the middle of a forest—truly an out-of-character place to find a BLM campground. A small river runs alongside the campsites here. Although fishless, it still provides a pleasant song for campers and plenty of inspiration for your imagination to create its own "Legend of the Lonesome Beaver" tale. No one seems to know the real story.

There are five sites here surrounded by tall trees you wouldn't typically associate with the Lake Powell area of Utah—among them Douglas-fir, spruce, ponderosa pine, and aspen. A bevy of smaller plant life also dots the landscape to add to the surprise of the Henries.

The fauna surrounding the area are perhaps what makes Lonesome Beaver so atypical. The Henry Mountains are the only place in the lower 48 states where you'll find a

Despite this campground's name, you'll probably spot more deer and turkeys around here than beavers.

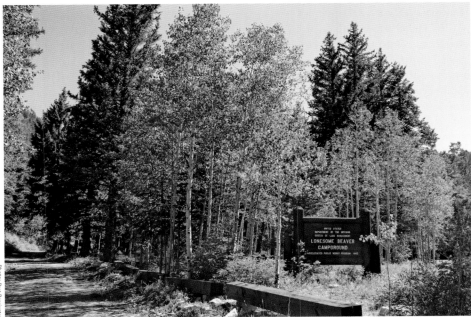

Photo: *Bret Remington*

KEY INFORMATION

LOCATION: Sawmill Basin Road, Hanksville, UT 84734

CONTACT: 435-542-3461, blm.gov/utah

OPERATED BY: Bureau of Land Management, Henry Mountains Field Station

OPEN: May–October

SITES: 5

EACH SITE: Picnic table, fire ring, barbecue stand

ASSIGNMENT: First-come, first-served; no reservations

REGISTRATION: On-site self-registration

AMENITIES: Vault toilets, drinking water

PARKING: At campsites only

FEE: $4/night

WHEELCHAIR ACCESS: Not designated

ELEVATION: 8,230'

RESTRICTIONS:

PETS: On leash only

FIRES: In fire rings only

ALCOHOL: Permitted

VEHICLES: No stated length limit, but a high-clearance four-wheel-drive vehicle is recommended for traveling the road to the campground.

OTHER: 14-day stay limit

---

free-roaming herd of American bison that are still hunted. The state issues a few dozen permits each year, so chances of getting a shot are slim. For better odds, talk to the Henry Mountains Field Office about where you might catch a peek at the herd and have a chance to shoot a few photos.

Mountain lions, mule deer, rabbits, and numerous bird species also call this unique place their home. When I arrived at the campground, it was full of wild turkeys. I counted more than 30, although it could have easily been more. (Have *you* ever tried counting a rafter of turkeys while they're riled up about the human thing chasing them with a camera? Not easy.)

The Henry Mountains seem to rise up out of the desert and beckon the adventurous traveler to come explore the outstretched fingers of its canyons. Geologists delight in the unique formation of the steep mountainside. It's believed that molten lava pushed its way upward but could not break the thick layer of earth crust. Instead, the crust only bulged without rupturing to create laccoliths—the five prominent peaks of the Henries. Over time, erosion has exposed the now-hardened diorite core of the mountain. Visitors can explore different areas of the mountain to see these formations and the transitions to more typical geology in the surrounding area.

One of the best ways to enjoy the Henry Mountains is to take the alternate route to the campground along Bull Mountain Road and over Wickiup Pass. Catch Bull Mountain Road off of UT 95, about 20 miles south of Hanksville. You'll climb steadily right up the mountainside, getting a chance to peer east over Glen Canyon National Recreation Area and driving through a massive burn area to see the power of fire up close and personal.

Bull Mountain Road was actually in better condition than Sawmill Basin Road on my visit, though heavy rains, winter damage, and maintenance schedules could affect that. Bring a high-clearance vehicle just to be sure.

Although not everyone signs in at the campground kiosk, it's noteworthy that I was just the fifth person to sign the camp register one year, and I made my visit *after* Labor Day when there was already snow in the peaks. You've got a good chance at some alone time here. Even the BLM doesn't make too many trips to the campground, so be extra-vigilant in maintaining and cleaning up your campsite.

Below the campground is the Dandelion Flats day-use area. It appears this picnic and play area is frequented more often than the campground, and would make an excellent day trip for anyone looking for a brief respite from the heat of nearby Lake Powell on their extended camping trip.

There are a few trails in the area for hiking enthusiasts. Visit Bull Mountain Pass and take the 4-mile trail to Mount Ellen. At 11,600 feet, you get spectacular views of the surrounding desert. Or, leave from Dandelion Flats and go 4 miles around Mount Ellen Ridge.

However you enjoy Lonesome Beaver, you'll be one of the few who has. With such a singular personality and unique geology, this is one campground that will call out to you until you come for a visit.

Lonesome Beaver Campground

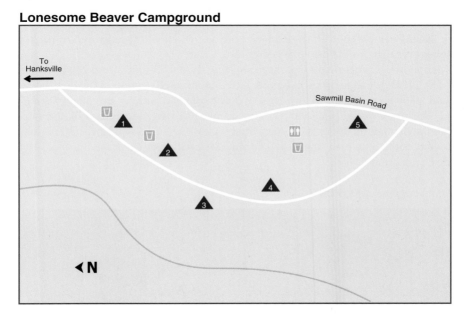

GETTING THERE

From the intersection of UT 24 and North 100 East in Hanksville, go 23 miles south on paved, then gravel, then dirt 100 East (Sawmill Basin Road) to the campground entrance, on your right.

GPS COORDINATES: N38° 6.577' W110° 46.688'

42

Moonflower Campground

Beauty: ★★★★★ / Privacy: ★★★★ / Quiet: ★★★★★ / Spaciousness: ★★★ / Security: ★★★★ /
Cleanliness: ★★★★★

Moonflower is a magical place. It's only 3 miles from Moab but seems like 300.

If adventure has a home address, you can bet it's got a Moab zip code. This town of 5,000 is the hub of activity in southeastern Utah. It's the headquarters of mountain biking, hiking, river running, and four-wheel drive exploration. Main Street Moab is like the Las Vegas Strip for outdoor addicts, with dozens of guides, outfitters, and gear rental shops. It's high-octane adventure within easy reach of high-calorie fast-food joints.

It's no wonder thousands of people flock to this town each year. It's an exciting place to be, but the constant buzz of activity can make you dizzy. How great it is then, to have a place like the campground at Moonflower Canyon to dull out the noise and recharge your batteries overnight for the next day's adventure.

Moonflower Campground is a magical place. It's only 3 miles from Moab but seems like 300. While Moab moves at a frantic pace, Moonflower remains oblivious. The campground follows a small and narrow canyon that begins at a parking area along Kane Creek Road. The massive sheer walls wrap around a small trail dotted with six walk-in campsites within the Behind the Rocks Wilderness Study Area. As you move deeper into the canyon, the noises of the busy road fade away, and you're left with only silence in the cool air of the shaded campground.

Shady spots abound at Moonflower.

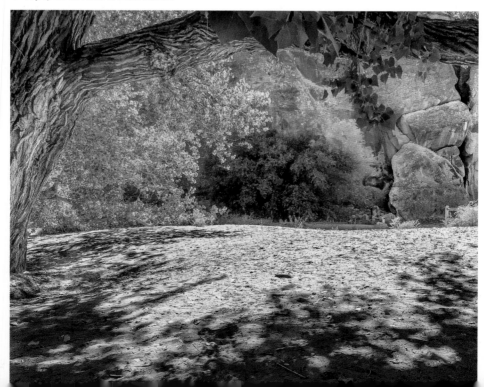

KEY INFORMATION

LOCATION: Kane Creek Boulevard west of Moab, UT 84532

CONTACTS: 435-259-2100, blm.gov/utah; reservations: 877-444-6777, recreation.gov

OPERATED BY: Bureau of Land Management, Moab Field Office

OPEN: Year-round

SITES: 6, plus 1 group site

EACH SITE: Fire ring

ASSIGNMENT: First-come, first-served; group site by reservation

REGISTRATION: On-site self-registration or online (group site)

FACILITIES: Vault toilets, garbage service

PARKING: In unpaved group lot

FEE: $10/night (single), $60/night (group)

WHEELCHAIR ACCESS: Restrooms only

ELEVATION: 5,842'

RESTRICTIONS:

PETS: On leash only

FIRES: In fire rings only

ALCOHOL: Permitted

VEHICLES: Up to 15 feet

OTHER: 14-day stay limit; maximum 10 people, 2 vehicles/per site (single) or 20 people, 10 vehicles/site (group)

Skip past sites 1–3 unless you're a heavy sleeper. Kane Creek Road always has plenty of traffic, and the engine sounds still reach those sites and bounce off the canyon walls. Instead, go deeper into the canyon to site 6, the undisputed jewel of the campground. Set far away from the other sites and out of earshot of the road, it'll make feel like you're in the middle of nowhere, as your tent is set underneath the trees and nestled against the canyon wall. Sites 4–8 are also nice but just a bit closer together than ideal.

There are other campgrounds along Kane Creek Road. The Bureau of Land Management (BLM) recently completed construction of more than 100 new sites at Ledge Campgrounds A–E, though they're very exposed to the elements. Rumor has it that the BLM is looking to convert Moonflower into a day-use-only site, but it was still open as of my last visit. If it does close, Hunter Canyon Campground, just a few more miles down the road, is a close second, or if you can nab one of the two sites at Spring Campground, it's a good third option. The BLM has tightened restrictions on dispersed camping all around Moab, so you need to either find an established campground for the night or get very familiar with the BLM's latest map showing restrictions (see discovermoab.com/campgrounds_blm.htm). It's no fun to get a figurative knock on your tent door in the morning from enforcement officers.

The best way to start your own adventure in Moab is to visit the city's information center, conveniently located on the southeast corner of Main and Center Streets in Moab. Here you'll find stands of free brochures ranging from public-land information to the obligatory "Please spend your money with us!" promotional materials. The knowledgeable staff can help you narrow down your choices to find the option that best suits you. There's also a small bookstore and gift shop. As you know, a great guidebook (ahem) is an invaluable tool when planning to use your valuable vacation days.

Just 5 miles farther up Kane Creek Boulevard from Moonflower Canyon is Hunters Canyon. From a small parking area, you can begin your exploration of this rugged canyon. Hunter Arch is a popular hiking destination. Although the arch itself isn't the biggest or most spectacular arch in the area, the hike through Navajo Sandstone is enjoyable and the destination notable.

One of the most popular activities for visitors to Moab is river rafting. The Colorado River can accommodate paddlers of all abilities, from kids to hardcore kayakers. There's no shortage of river guides, but tours can fill up quickly so it's best to book ahead. Visit discovermoab.com for more information about local guides and outfitters.

Moab is also world-renowned for its mountain biking. The most talked-about trail in town is the Slickrock Trail, and with good reason. This 10.5-mile loop trail over sandstone opens at its peak to reveal a staggering view of the Colorado River. It can be rough in spots, requiring riders to be in good physical shape. If you're a little rusty (or if your bike is, for that matter), you may want to take the 2-mile practice loop before heading out on the actual trail. To get to the Slickrock Trail, go east on 300 South in Moab; turn right when the road ends, and then make a second left. You'll enter Sand Flats Recreation Area, where you'll have to pay a $5 day-use fee, and then go about a half mile to the trailhead.

When you come to Moab, bring your sense of adventure and plenty of ibuprofen. There are more adventures here than you could fulfill in a lifetime, and no better place to start them than from the quiet and magical Moonflower Campground.

Moonflower Campground

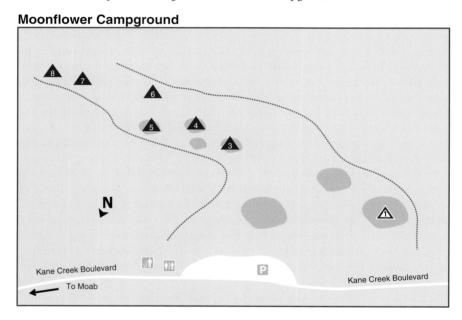

GETTING THERE

From I-70/US 6, take Exit 182 in Crescent Junction and drive south to Moab on US 191. After 32 miles, turn right at the Burger King onto Kane Creek Boulevard, and drive 3 miles to the campground, on your right.

GPS COORDINATES: N38° 33.251' W109° 35.225'

43

⛺ Natural Bridges National Monument Campground

Beauty: ★★★ / Privacy: ★★★ / Quiet: ★★★ / Spaciousness: ★★★★ / Security: ★★★★ / Cleanliness: ★★★★

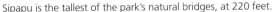

Kachina Bridge could fit the Great Sphinx or the Mayflower's top mast under her span.

Somewhere between the tiny town of Blanding and the recreation hot spot of Lake Powell lies the tiny little desert isle of Natural Bridges National Monument. The park encompasses just 7,636 acres, but each one holds something special that's just begging to be discovered.

Only about 125,000 people visit Natural Bridges each year, so the campground within the park is actually a great place to spend the night. That might seem like a lot of visitors, but when you consider that more than a half million people go to Canyonlands and 2.5 million see Glen Canyon each year, you've got an underutilized facility at your disposal.

The park's 13 campsites provide the essentials: a table and a place to set up your tent. There's no water on-site, but water and modern restrooms are available at the visitor center, less than a quarter mile away on a footpath that leaves directly from the campground. Garbage and recycling services *are* provided, so if Natural Bridges is one stop on your Tour de Southern Utah, you can unload your empties here with a clean conscience. The park is actually very eco-friendly: it runs on solar power collected from an array that's on display for public viewing.

Site 5 is probably the belle of the ball here, with sites 1–4 and 6 her runners-up. Avoid sites 7–9; they're a bit crammed in and more open to the scorching sun. Although the campground is open all year, summers can sizzle this far south. Come during fall, spring, or even winter to avoid a nasty sunburn and a sweat-soaked sleepless night.

Sipapu is the tallest of the park's natural bridges, at 220 feet.

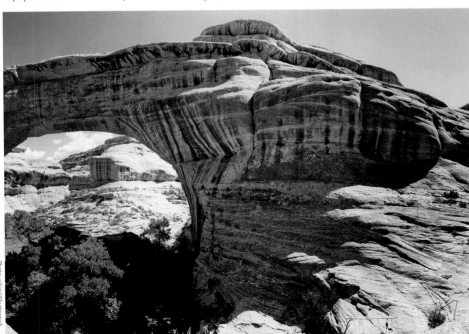

KEY INFORMATION

LOCATION: UT 275, Lake Powell, UT 84533

CONTACT: 435-692-1234, nps.gov/nabr

OPERATED BY: Natural Bridges National Monument, National Park Service

OPEN: Year-round

SITES: 13

EACH SITE: Picnic table, barbecue stand, tent pad

ASSIGNMENT: First-come, first-served; no reservations

REGISTRATION: On-site self-registration

AMENITIES: Vault toilets, garbage service, recycling; water and full restrooms 0.25 mile away at visitor center

PARKING: At campsites only

FEE: $10/night

WHEELCHAIR ACCESS: Campground is generally barrier-free but not officially ADA-accessible except for restrooms.

ELEVATION: 7,379'

RESTRICTIONS:

PETS: On leash only; prohibited on hiking trails

FIRES: In grills only

ALCOHOL: Permitted

VEHICLES: Up to 26 feet

OTHER: Maximum 8 people, 1 vehicle/site; water at visitor center limited to 5 gallons/person

All sites are first-come, first-served. If you can't get a spot, overflow camping is available back at the junction of UT 95 and UT 261; there's also dispersed camping along Deer Flats and Bear's Ears Roads. Camping along UT 275 is prohibited. Nearly all of the land surrounding the park is administered by the federal Bureau of Land Management, with the exception of the Abajo Mountains to the northeast, which lie within U.S. Forest Service land and hold their very own allure.

The park gets its name from three significant natural bridges: Sipapu, at 220 feet tall; Owachomo, at 210 feet; and Kachina, measuring 106 feet. To give you some perspective, the park once distributed a flyer comparing the heights of these bridges with those of other famous landmarks. The Statue of Liberty, from the top of the torch to the bottom of her feet, would fit underneath both Sipapu and Owachomo, with about 60 feet to spare. The Taj Mahal would also fit beneath these two bridges. Kachina Bridge could fit the Great Sphinx or the *Mayflower*'s top mast under her span, with 20 or 30 feet of breathing room. Only Rainbow Bridge, to the southeast near Lake Powell, can best these three bridges: the US Capitol could squeeze just underneath that 290-foot behemoth.

That all sounds dandy on paper, but you can't truly grasp how big the bridges are until you see them in person. Luckily, the park is set up for you to do just that. The park's main road, Bridge View Drive, turns into a one-way loop just past the campground. Rangers advise setting aside an hour or so to make the 9-mile circle; that leaves you with time to stop at each bridge's view area to snap a few pictures.

To get the full effect of these expansive natural formations, created by the scouring erosion of moving water over vast lengths of time, get out of the car and walk to the base of each bridge. The longest hike is 1.5 miles round-trip, so you won't have to dedicate a major portion of your day to each one. The routes are moderately strenuous, however; each will require you to hike over uneven steps, and both Kachina and Sipapu employ handrails and ladders.

Foot trails also connect the bridges for more-adventurous hikers, or you may opt to explore Horse Collar Ruin. This ancestral Puebloan site is believed to have been abandoned about 700 years ago, but it's remarkably well preserved—a real-life lesson in ancient architecture. Take the advice of park officials and pack at least 1 gallon of water per person, per day. Disturbing the ruins or climbing on the bridges themselves is, of course, prohibited.

Too many tourists pass Natural Bridges National Monument on their way to or coming back from somewhere. Don't be one of them. Plan on taking a detour and spending the night to marvel at some of the most impressive natural wonders in the world.

Natural Bridges National Monument Campground

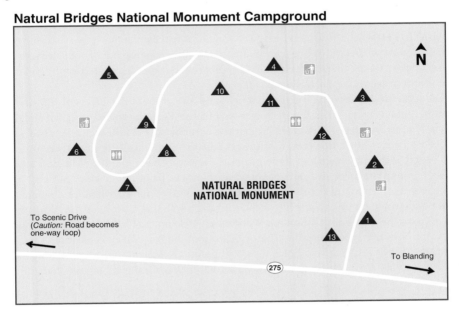

GETTING THERE

From the intersection of UT 95 and US 191 just south of Blanding, drive 30 miles west on UT 95; then turn right (west) onto UT 275 and drive 5 more miles to the campground entrance, on your right about 1 mile past the park gates.

GPS COORDINATES: N37° 36.526' W109° 59.004'

44

⛺ Oak Grove Campground

Beauty: ★★★★★ / Privacy: ★★★★ / Quiet: ★★★★ / Spaciousness: ★★★★ / Security: ★★★★★ /
Cleanliness: ★★★★★

Oak Grove moves at a slower pace than the other Pine Valley campgrounds.

Have you ever taken a long drive up a hot and dusty road and feared what you'd find at the end? Isn't it great when the drive pays off and you find a spectacular new place that you never even dreamed could exist? While it's a shame to take the suspense out of your drive to Oak Grove, I have to share that this hidden little campground is an unexpected happy ending to what first appeared an unpromising journey.

The road to Oak Grove will give you a firsthand lesson about the effects of elevation on plant life. After leaving Leeds and the tiny town of Silver Reef, the landscape is tan and drab, with only a few freckles of dark green juniper and scrubby sage. As the dusty dirt road winds farther up Leeds Creek, however, wildflowers appear—sporadically at first, then in profusion—and the journey begins to show promise. Flowering cacti line the road, and the fold of earth around the creek is a verdant vein that shimmies from side to side with each bend in the riverbed. As you near the campground, the oak trees appear. Then, as if on cue, the great ponderosa pine trees come into sight, forming a wall that surrounds the campground and protects the Pine Valley Mountain Wilderness. Welcome to Oak Grove Campground.

As the crow flies, you're now less than 4 miles from the Pine Valley Recreation Area. This U.S. Forest Service (USFS) land holds three campgrounds, a picnic area, and the small Pine Valley Reservoir. The problem is, you've got a 3,500-foot vertical cliff between you and that

A peek at a peak through the ponderosa pines

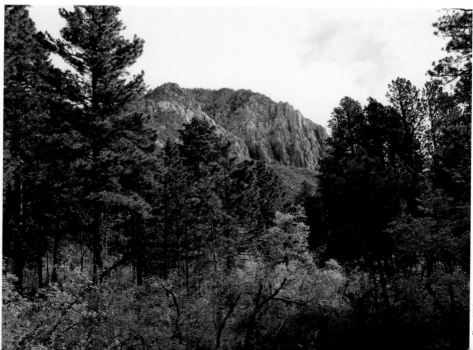

Photo: J. V. Remsen

KEY INFORMATION

LOCATION: FR 032, Pine Valley, UT 84781

CONTACT: 435-652-3100, tinyurl.com
/dixienfcamp

OPERATED BY: Dixie National Forest,
Pine Valley Ranger District

OPEN: Mid-May–October (depending
on weather)

SITES: 8 (including 1 double)

EACH SITE: Picnic table, fire ring,
barbecue stand

ASSIGNMENT: First-come, first-served;
no reservations

REGISTRATION: On-site self-registration

AMENITIES: Vault toilets, drinking water

PARKING: At campsites or day-use lot

FEE: $5/night

WHEELCHAIR ACCESS: Not designated

ELEVATION: 6,380'

RESTRICTIONS:

PETS: On leash only

FIRES: In fire rings only

ALCOHOL: Permitted

VEHICLES: RVs and trailers not recommended
due to narrow access road

OTHER: 14-day stay limit

---

recreation complex. You'll soon come to realize that the cliff isn't really a problem at all—rather a blessed buffer between you and the many OHVs, trailers, and constant drone of activity up on top. Oak Grove moves at a slower pace than the other Pine Valley campgrounds.

If you decide that you do want to go check out the recreation area on foot, you'll have to work to get there. Take the Oak Grove Trail from the trailhead in camp, and you'll make your way up a steep incline, then around the side of the cliffs before mounting a straight ascent on the Browns Point Trail. You'll have views of Zion National Park and even northern Arizona from this 6-mile trail, but every snapshot will be paid for with your burning legs and heavy breathing. Considering, however, that the drive would force you to go all the way around the mountain and take over an hour and a half, foot-powered exploration is a viable option.

With more than 50,000 acres under the federal wilderness designation, you've got plenty of hikes to choose from. The Summit Trail follows the backbone of the Pine Valley Mountains for 18 miles, or you can bag Washington County's highest peak, Signal Peak, at 10,365 feet.

The campsites at Oak Grove provide enough space and privacy to keep you happy, except perhaps sites 4–6. Double site 5 is planted on the side of the road where the line between road, parking lot, and campsite becomes blurred. Still, the campground is quiet enough that even these sites are OK. Set up camp in site 1 to stay away from the other sites. You'll have to hoof it to the parking area by site 2 for water, but the privacy is worth the sacrifice. Site 8, also removed from the rest, has a mysterious wooden gazebo nearby. Exactly why a wooden gazebo sits at the edge of the campground is never explained, but it is a nice bonus feature, especially if you're camping with somebody you love.

Indeed, this campground is something of an enigma. While it's clearly noted on USFS and online maps and it even has Yelp reviews, it's not in the master campground list at Dixie National Forest's official website.

Note that Oak Grove isn't immune from off-road vehicles. Back down the dirt road toward town, they've left their mark and are a popular place for locals to pull back on the throttle. According to USFS rules, however, they can't be ridden inside the campground boundaries, and above the camp is designated wilderness where they are strictly forbidden.

Fishing opportunities are pretty scant in this neck of the woods. Leeds Creek holds a small population of native Bonneville cutthroats, which were actually transplanted from the other side of the mountain. Tributaries to Leeds Creek, including Pig Creek, Horse Creek, and Spirit Creek, are also accessible by foot and contain some of the small trout. Practice catching and releasing in these waters to help sustain the precious population of Bonnies.

Oak Grove is on the doorstep of Utah's second-largest wilderness area, yet your chances of being alone here are extremely high. The Pine Valley Mountains beckon you to explore their unsung trails and rugged beauty. Discover a new favorite camping spot, drink from a refreshingly cold spring, and take advantage of all that Oak Grove has to offer.

Oak Grove Campground

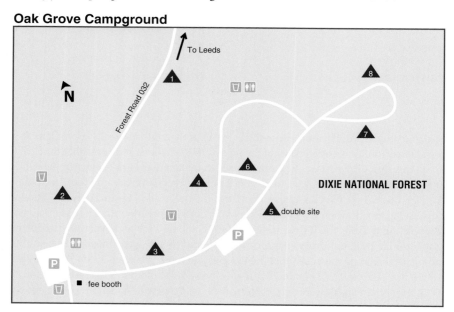

GETTING THERE

From I-15, take eastbound Exit 22 (16 miles northwest of St. George) or westbound Exit 23 (286 miles south of Salt Lake City) in Leeds, and drive northwest on Silver Reef Road, which becomes dirt Forest Road 032. In 3.1 miles, bear right at the fork to continue north on FR 032. Follow the road 5.6 miles to its end; the campground is just across Leeds Creek.

GPS COORDINATES: N37° 19.049' W113° 27.079'

45

Oowah Lake Campground

Beauty: ★★★★★ / Privacy: ★★★★ / Quiet: ★★★★ / Spaciousness: ★★★ / Security: ★★★★ /
Cleanliness: ★★★★

This campground is a refuge from the blazing sun of the valley below.

It's a strange name for a campground. Is it a Native American tribal name? Nope. A foreign word given by immigrant settlers? Uh-uh. Take a moment to say it: *Oowah. Ooh. Aah.* That's the sound you'll make when you reach this heaven on high.

I frequently have to make the case that Oowah Campground is a real place. After all, it's only about 40 minutes from downtown Moab, which conjures up images of red rock, desert, and sky-high temperatures. But this oasis is very real, indeed. It's an honest-to-goodness forest of the La Sal Mountains on the southeast side of town, and the campground is a refuge from the blazing sun of the valley below.

There are two routes to the campground, but both will probably be the reason for your first oohs and aahs. Either drive south from Moab on US 191 and take the turn for Old Airport Road and make your way up La Sal Loop Road, or head north out of town to the Colorado River. From there, you'll go upriver on UT 128 some 15 miles before turning toward Castle Valley and winding up the mountain. The southern route is faster, but the Castle

The scenery at Oowah Lake will have you oohing and aahing for real.

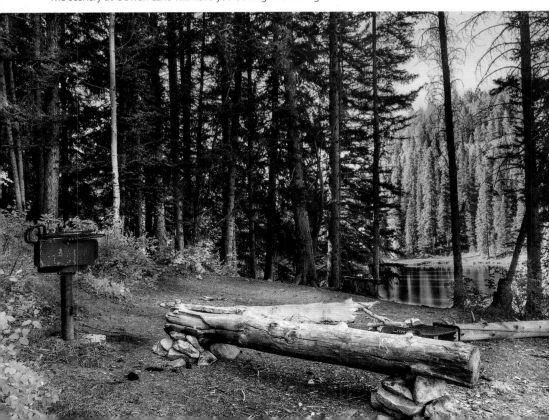

KEY INFORMATION

LOCATION: FR 0076, Moab, UT 84532

CONTACT: 435-259-7155, tinyurl.com
/mantilasalcamping

OPERATED BY: Manti–La Sal National Forest,
Moab Ranger District

OPEN: Mid-May–mid-October

SITES: 11

EACH SITE: Picnic table, fire ring, barbecue
stand

ASSIGNMENT: First-come, first-served;
no reservations

REGISTRATION: On-site self-registration

AMENITIES: Vault toilets, picnic area

PARKING: Group lot

FEE: $5/night

WHEELCHAIR ACCESS: Accessible restroom

ELEVATION: 8,800'

RESTRICTIONS:

PETS: On leash only

FIRES: In fire rings only

ALCOHOL: Permitted

VEHICLES: No stated length limit

OTHER: 14-day stay limit

Valley way will leave your breathless, with views of spires, buttes, and the winding Colorado River below, especially when driven from the campground down on the way home.

If that doesn't have you cooing in approval, you'll certainly see why the name fits when you arrive at Oowah Lake and Campground. The glassy waters of the tiny lake tumble down the other side of the dam and create that special gurgling soundtrack that only a small stream can provide. Thick forest surrounds the waters, and if you listen closely, you can hear the sounds of small trout smacking the surface as they lap up flies.

There are 11 campsites here, along with a large group day-use area. Three of the sites sit below the main parking area and back up into the river—albeit at a safe distance—while sites 4 and 5 are walk-in only and are perched above the lake. Choose one of those two if you want to be near the water, but recognize that the trail around the lake passes directly by your sites.

The rest of the sites are along a road that rises gently away from the parking spots and have a small needle eye loop at the end. Site 11 is at the end of the loop and the least spacious or private, while site 6 is large but exposed. Tenters will delight in any of the sites from 7 to 10. There are two sets of restrooms available, the newer set being wheelchair-accessible.

In several visits to Oowah, there's one thing I don't encounter much, and that's people. In spring, I found brilliant blue, orange, and yellow butterflies, but no humans. In the 110-degree heat of summer, I escaped the swelter and only found three cars in the parking lot. After Labor Day, I found an empty campground on a Friday night. Even the kind forest ranger I asked told me that on weekends in the height of the summer, it's not uncommon to find the campground with only four or five sites occupied. Ooh and ahh as loudly as you'd like, and you may not wake your neighbors.

Don't think that the La Sal Mountains are just an out-of-the-way stop for national-park visitors, though. The small pocket of mountains in this region holds its own as a recreational destination. Hiking, biking, fishing, and scenic drives make the La Sals a unique and rewarding place.

From camp, there's a loop hike to Clark Lake. Leave across the dam or around the east side of the lake, and climb 700 feet for a 3-mile endeavor. Or take the 1.5-mile uphill trek to

Warner Lake and the campground there (a good alternative if Oowah were to ever fill up) and there are hikes to Miners Basin (2 miles), Burro Pass (4 miles), and the Dry Fork–Beaver Basin Trail (5 miles).

Autumn in the La Sals is especially brilliant. The radiant yellow leaves of the aspens look like paint strokes on the canvas of the canyon slopes. This spectacular show is idyllic for any fall-loving photographer.

If summer is the only time you can get away to Canyonlands or Arches, sneak up the mountains. It's worth the extra time driving to sleep sweatless, but don't overlook the La Sals as a destination in their own right. There's certainly plenty here to keep you oohing and ahhing time and time again.

Oowah Lake Campground

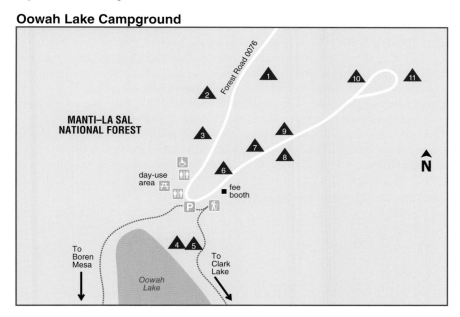

GETTING THERE

From I-70/US 6, take Exit 182 in Crescent Junction and drive south on US 191, passing through Moab. After 39 miles, turn left onto Old Airport Road in Spanish Valley; in 0.6 mile, turn right onto Spanish Valley Drive, which becomes La Sal Loop Road. In 9 miles, bear left at the intersection to stay on this road. In another 0.8 mile, keep straight at a second intersection and, in another 0.7 mile, bear right at a third intersection to continue on La Sal Loop Road. In 2.4 miles, La Sal Loop Road veers left—continue straight, now on Forest Road 0076, and follow it another 3 miles to the campground, at the end of FR 0076 shortly after you cross Mill Creek.

GPS COORDINATES: N38° 30.12' W109° 16.392'

46

Pleasant Creek Campground

Beauty: ★★★★★ / Privacy: ★★★ / Quiet: ★★★ / Spaciousness: ★★★★ / Security: ★★★ /
Cleanliness: ★★★★

Pleasant Creek is the best place to stay on Boulder Mountain.

It would be wrong to say that Boulder Mountain is in the middle of nowhere. On the contrary, this magnificent and rugged part of Dixie National Forest is in the middle of everything, and Pleasant Creek is the best place to stay on Boulder Mountain. (While the campground is within Dixie National Forest, it's administered by Fishlake National Forest.)

A quick calculation by a popular online mapping service shows the drive time to the town of Torrey at 3 hours and 44 minutes from the biggest cities of both Salt Lake and Washington Counties, the most populated counties of northern and southern Utah, respectively. That means that most Utahns could leave work on a Friday afternoon and be sitting in a camp chair listening to the bubbling waters of Pleasant Creek as it passes by their tent just as the summer sun goes down. Campers from farther away may have to ditch the last hour of work, but that's what Friday afternoons are all about . . . right?

Pleasant Creek is actually split between two separate campgrounds: upper and lower. The upper is spread around an open loop, with each site's parking plot spurred from the main circle. There are 12 first-come, first-served sites surrounded by tall pines reached

Pleasant Creek overlooks Capitol Reef National Park.

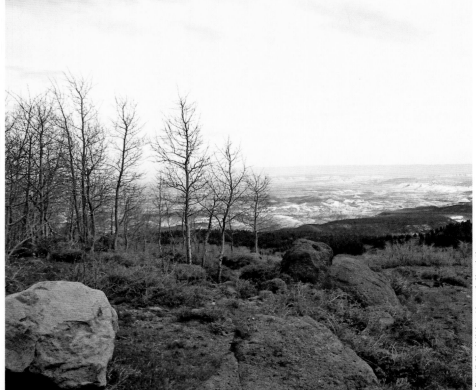

KEY INFORMATION

LOCATION: UT 12, Teasdale, UT 84772

CONTACTS: 435-836-2800, tinyurl.com/fishlakenfcamping

OPERATED BY: High Country Recreation for Fishlake National Forest, Fremont River Ranger District

OPEN: Mid-May–mid-October, depending on weather

SITES: 16

EACH SITE: Picnic table, fire ring

ASSIGNMENT: First-come, first-served; no reservations

REGISTRATION: On-site self-registration at lower campground

AMENITIES: Vault toilets, drinking water

PARKING: At campsites only

FEES: $10/night, $5/additional vehicle

WHEELCHAIR ACCESS: Site 4

ELEVATION: 8,750'

RESTRICTIONS:

PETS: On leash only

FIRES: In fire rings only

ALCOHOL: Permitted

VEHICLES: Up to 25 feet

OTHER: 14-day stay limit

by crossing Pleasant Creek. Site 4 is ADA-accessible, and garbage service is provided throughout.

At the lower campground, things are a bit more intimate. There are only five sites here, and they back into Pleasant Creek as it turns away from the highway on its way to delivering water into Lower Bowns Reservoir. The campsites fit snugly together around a shorter loop and are each allotted a bit less space than are the upper sites.

You probably won't encounter any RVs at the lower site. A sign at the entrance advises against them. According to the site host, most RVs actually fly by Pleasant Creek in favor of other nearby campgrounds like Singletree or Lower Bowns, which are bigger and more accommodating to RV needs. If Pleasant Creek happens to be full, try Oak Creek Campground as a backup, just over a mile south on UT 12. It too caters to tent campers.

It's hard to get locals to talk about "The Boulder." They're fiercely protective of the high-mountain retreat. Perhaps that's why it's rarely visited by anyone but locals and coincidental passersby. Try to pry a favorite fishing hole out of a Boulder Mountain regular, and you'd think you were asking for their private bank account number. They're tight-lipped for a reason; some of the biggest brook trout in the state swim in the dozens of lakes on the mountain. The state record brookie, a 7-pound, 8-ounce beast, was caught here in 1971, and the record still stands today. You may just have to buy a topographical map and start exploring all the blue dots. Don't overlook the thin blue lines, though: in addition to holding some great brook and cut-throat trout, the rivers here will lead you to some picture-perfect places, where the elements of a model forest—blue skies, clear water, towering trees—all come together before your eyes.

If you're feeling adventurous, take a drive to the Aquarius Plateau, or "Boulder Top," as it's more commonly known. Be forewarned, however, that the Boulders are appropriately named. What can look like an innocent dirt road to begin with quickly turns into a gnarly, menacing 4x4 experience. These roads are unrepentant in their desire to eat your truck and leave you stranded. High-clearance four-wheel-drive vehicles are absolutely required on all off-road excursions.

To reach Boulder Top, you'll (1) have to drive to the town of Bicknell and take Posey Lake Road and Forest Road 178 south, or (2) drive all the way back down to Escalante and follow the signs north on FR 153 to Posey Lake Campground. These roads are typically closed until the middle of June because of snow, so call the U.S. Forest Service ahead of time to check conditions. If you've braved the rough roads, you'll find enough hiking and fishing on the Aquarius Plateau to keep you coming back for years.

Stay near camp at Pleasant Creek, and you'll still have plenty of places to drown a worm on a hook. Lower Bowns Reservoir, just a jog from Pleasant Creek Campground, is stocked with always-willing rainbow and tiger trout, and many brook trout find their way in from the surrounding tributaries. Within a few minutes' drive, you can access the trail to Oak Creek Reservoir and nearby Round, Scout, and Long Lakes. Farther south still on UT 12 is the trail to Deer Creek Lake and Green, Moosman, and Steep Creek Lakes. There are too many lakes to name, too many trails to detail. Trial and error never sounds so fun as it does here on Boulder Mountain.

It's easy to get into a camping rut going to the same campgrounds month after month, year after year. There's a simple antidote for same-site syndrome: pack up the gear and point your car toward Boulder Mountain. It's closer than you think.

Pleasant Creek Campground

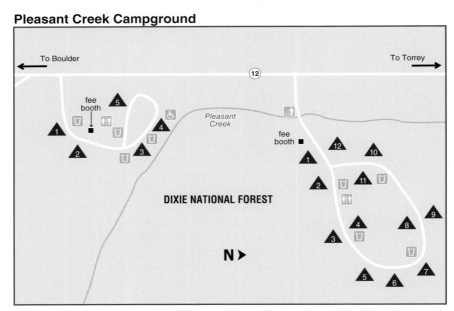

GETTING THERE

From the intersection of UT 12 and UT 24 in Torrey, drive 17 miles south on UT 12 to the signed campground entrance, on your left.

GPS COORDINATES: N38° 6.043' W111° 20.188'

47

⛺ Red Cliffs Campground

Beauty: ★★★★★ / Privacy: ★★★★ / Quiet: ★★★ / Spaciousness: ★★★★ / Security: ★★★★ /
Cleanliness: ★★★★

Start your adventure exploring a magnificent desert reserve from Red Cliffs Campground.

In 1996 an impressive coalition of federal and state land managers, cities, environmental groups, and local counties realized the need to protect the fragile ecosystem of southwestern Utah, so they united to create the Red Cliffs Desert Reserve. Some 62,000 acres were set aside to protect animals like the desert tortoise—federally listed as threatened—and other varieties of wildlife on the state's Sensitive Species List of animals that have become increasingly pressured by rapid population growth and heightened recreational land use.

Today, the reserve represents a magnificent opportunity for some of the best desert camping and hiking in the state. Start your adventure by staying at Red Cliffs Campground. It's the ideal place to get hydrated and rest up for a day of desert hiking.

Although temperatures in the reserve can soar well above 100°F in the summer, you'll find some relief at Red Cliffs. Tiny Quail Creek (sometimes referred to as Harrisburg Creek) trickles down through the campground most days, providing just enough moisture for a thriving population of giant cottonwoods along the banks. These trees and the protective red cliffs of the campground's namesake are enough to take the edge off of oppressive summer heat. The canyon walls also keep the winds down, making the campground a superb place to plan a camping trip when the rest of the state is just too cold. Beware of sudden rainstorms, though, as the creek can rise dramatically with just a few minutes of intense rain, rendering the road back to town impassable.

Hikers explore Red Cliffs Desert Reserve.

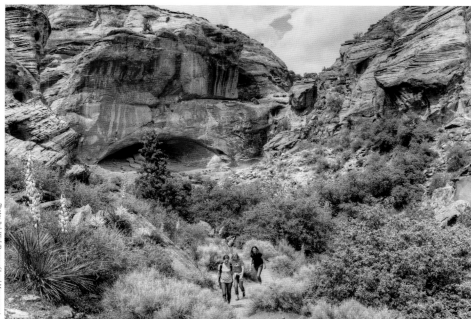

KEY INFORMATION

LOCATION: North of I-15, Hurricane, UT 84737

CONTACT: 435-688-3200, blm.gov/utah

OPERATED BY: Bureau of Land Management, St. George Field Office

OPEN: Year-round

SITES: 11

EACH SITE: Picnic table, fire ring, barbecue stand

ASSIGNMENT: First-come, first-served; no reservations

REGISTRATION: On-site self-registration

AMENITIES: Vault toilets, drinking water, garbage service, picnic areas

PARKING: At campsites or in day-use lot

FEE: $15/night

WHEELCHAIR ACCESS: Sites 8 and 11; accessible restrooms

ELEVATION: 3,120'

RESTRICTIONS:

PETS: On leash only

FIRES: In fire rings only

ALCOHOL: Permitted

VEHICLES: Up to 25 feet

OTHER: 14-day stay limit; wood gathering prohibited

Scattered under the cottonwoods alongside the campground's main road loop are 11 typical Bureau of Land Management campsites, each with a table, fire ring, and barbecue stand. Nearly all of the sites also have a shade awning over the picnic table, as trees are rare around the actual tent sites. One of the real pluses of this campground is the availability of drinking water. Spigots are generously placed over the grounds ensuring that you never have to walk far to fill your canteen.

Most sites here are equal, with a pull-in spur, a table, an awning, and precious little flora. To get as far as you can from the other campers, pick site 1 or 2. Sites 3 and 4 are crammed a little too close together for my liking but would work well for a large group that needed to split between two sites. Numbers 8 and 11 accommodate campers with disabilities, as do the vault toilets.

Three trails leave from the campground. The Silver Reef Trail is a short uphill jaunt leading to the overlook of an area where silver was mined in the early 1900s. The half-mile interpretive trail will help you identify the plant species around you, and the Red Cliffs Village Trail takes you to an old Anasazi ruin dating back to 1000 A.D. Each trail is easy to hike, even for young children, but both close at sunset.

For more-adventurous hikes, head into the Red Cliffs Desert Reserve, accessible near the campground on the road back to town. The boundaries are clearly marked and you'll know when you've reached the reserve's edge. "Step-overs" placed at entrances to the reserve are not only physical reminders of the special land designation but mental reminders of the special hiking, biking, and equestrian regulations. By crossing a step-over, visitors also acknowledge their responsibility to help protect the fragile desert ecology by not interfering with the wildlife. For more information on specific regulations, see redcliffsdesertreserve.com.

The reserve sits at the crossroads of three distinct ecosystems—the Mojave Desert, Great Basin, and Colorado Plateau—giving the land here an eclectic collection of inhabitants like the desert tortoise, Gila monster, chuckwalla, and sidewinder rattlesnake. One hundred ten species of reptiles, mammals, amphibians, and birds are found here, several dozen of which are considered sensitive and some of which are known to exist only in this area. Be mindful of your surroundings, and be especially vigilant to look out for venomous snakes in the area. Most won't bother you unless provoked—but snakes have little interest in discerning if your provocation was on purpose or by accident.

The flora of Red Cliffs are also a hodgepodge of plant life from three different ecosystems. Look for a healthy population of blackbrush, more commonly found in cooler climates, or one of the species of yucca and cacti that flourish at Red Cliffs. You'll also have a good chance to snap a photo of Utah's official state flower, the sego lily.

Serious hikers will appreciate the convenience of Red Cliffs, families will enjoy the picnic-like atmosphere of its shady river bottom, and anyone will welcome the shelter this campground provides during both the hottest and coldest Utah months.

Red Cliffs Campground

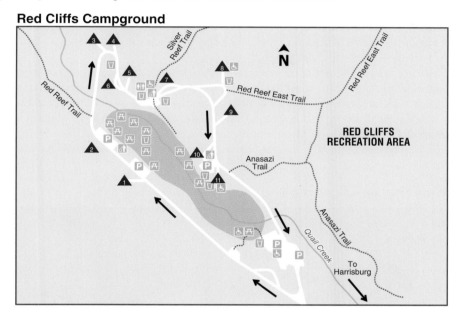

GETTING THERE

From I-15, take eastbound Exit 22 in Leeds, and go southwest on Old Highway 91 to the town of Harrisburg; from westbound Exit 23, turn left onto Silver Reef Road and then right onto Main Street, and drive 1.6 miles to merge onto Old Highway 91. In 2 miles, turn right just after the brown signs for Red Cliffs National Conservation Area and Red Cliffs Recreation Area. Go west under the freeway, take the first left, and then drive another 1.5 miles north to the entrance of Red Cliffs Recreation Area and the campground.

GPS COORDINATES: N37° 13.380' W113° 24.240'

48

Snow Canyon State Park Campground

Beauty: ★★★★ / Privacy: ★★★ / Quiet: ★★★ / Spaciousness: ★★★ / Security: ★★★ / Cleanliness: ★★★★★

When the winter blues become insufferable, book a site and get camping!

In a state where there are sometimes only two seasons—winter and August—Snow Canyon State Park is a little piece of heaven. When the winter blues become insufferable, book a site and get camping!

Less than 15 miles from the Arizona border, Snow Canyon encompasses just more than 5,700 acres of dramatic rolling canyons, which can vary in color from very deep, dark reds, to hues of tan, gold, and even white. Crowning large areas of this colored Navajo sandstone are large, twisted veins of black lava rock formed by three separate episodes of ancient volcanic activity.

In spite of its name, Snow Canyon rarely sees any snow, so it's an ideal place to go when other campgrounds are snowed in or just too cold. Temperatures can dip at night during the colder months, but it's the daytime weather that attracts the crowds. A good sleeping bag and a knit beanie will probably do the trick to get you through the night, although you'll probably want to get up and get moving early. Most campsites are shaded for a long time in the morning due to their location against the large, rounded stone cliffs that serve the campground's backdrop.

A desert red-rock tableau at Snow Canyon

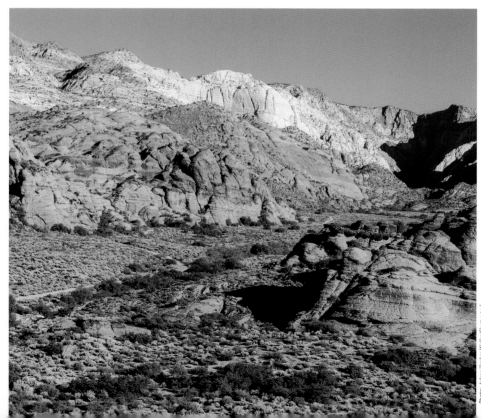

KEY INFORMATION

LOCATION: Snow Canyon Road off UT 18, Ivins, UT 84738

CONTACTS: 435-628-2255, stateparks.utah .gov/parks/snow-canyon; reservations: 800-322-3770, reserveamerica.com

OPERATED BY: Snow Canyon State Park

OPEN: Year-round

SITES: 31, plus 2 group sites

EACH SITE: Picnic table, fire ring, barbecue stand

ASSIGNMENT: First-come, first-served or by reservation

REGISTRATION: On-site self-registration or online

AMENITIES: Flush toilets, drinking water, garbage service, showers

PARKING: At campsites only

FEES: $20/night (single, nonelectric), $25/ night (single, electric), $75/night (Cottontail group site), $100/night (Quail group site), $10/additional vehicle (non-electric), $13/additional vehicle (electric); $6 park entrance fee

WHEELCHAIR ACCESS: Sites 1–14, restrooms

ELEVATION: 3,400'

RESTRICTIONS:

PETS: Permitted on leash only in campground, on West Canyon Road, and on Whiptail Trail

FIRES: In fire rings only; wood burning prohibited June 1–September 15 (charcoal and propane permitted)

ALCOHOL: Permitted

VEHICLES: Up to 40 feet

OTHER: 5-day stay limit; maximum 8 people/ site (single), 35 people/site (Cottontail), or 50 people/site (Quail); tents on pads only

The campground is more or less a large figure-eight pressed up against the side of a sandstone cliff. Turn in from the main park road and you'll immediately see the park office; continue to your right for sites 1–19 or to your left for the quieter sites, 20–29.

Sites 1–4 and 8–17 are set aside for RV use only. These sites resemble a drive-through more than a campsite, but suit RVers who are looking for a place to park and be hooked up. These RV sites remain isolated from the individual tent sites located on both ends of the figure-eight and quickly blend in with other structures near the campground entrance. Sites 20–21, 24, and 26–27 are the only sites assigned on a first-come, first-served basis. In addition to the 31 individual sites, there are two group sites: Quail holds 50, and Cottontail holds 35. Each can be reserved for $75 per night.

The tent sites here are liberally spaced and, wherever possible, inserted among the trees and high shrubbery to allow for the most privacy. In particular, sites 17, 20–22, and 26–29 will keep you sheltered from the views of others and enhance your outdoors experience. Showers and modern restrooms are available, so you won't completely escape the modern world. But just being outdoors in the middle of January or February will unquestionably feel good regardless.

Although much of the park's focus is directed on all the different kinds of rocks, lava flows, and unique park geology, the campground itself has plenty of smooth sand where you can set up a tent and sleep comfortably. You may want to build a roaring fire to keep warm during the cold desert night, but check with officials about current fire restrictions. Drought and fear of devastating wildfire have led to the prohibition of fires from June through the middle of September in recent years.

The same volcanic activity that deposited black and gray rock flows also left the park with lava tubes and caves that beg to be explored. The Butterfly Trail is a moderate 2-mile trail that leads to West Canyon Overlook and some of the park's famous lava tubes. Exploring any lava tubes or caves can be risky business, so use good judgment and always err on the side of caution.

For a slightly less intimidating hike, take the Pioneer Names Trail. When pioneers came through Snow Canyon in the late 1800s, some stopped to write their names in axle grease. Their names remain on the sandstone face, some dating back to 1883. The half-mile trail is relatively level and takes you right to the pioneer autographs.

Most trails are open to hikers, bikers, and horsemen alike. Rock climbing, however, has become a large part of the recreation in the park. Park officials ask that visitors not climb the rocks behind the campground and instead seek approved places to scale the sandstone. If you're new to climbing, a local outfitter conducts technical climbing classes in the park. Check with a park ranger for details about climbing classes and current climbing regulations.

Don't think that the cold months are the only time to come to Snow Canyon. If you want to explore and avoid the biggest crowds, July and August are sure to meet your needs. Temps often reach above 100°F and only slip to 70°F at night, but you'll find a little more breathing room than you normally would in April or October.

While your neighbors are sitting at home for another winter evening full of sappy primetime TV and stuffy recirculated air, stay at Snow Canyon State Park and camp when you never thought it was possible.

Snow Canyon State Park Campground

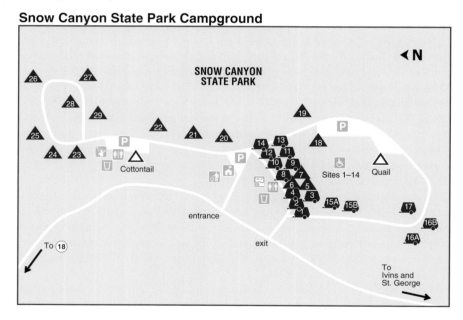

GETTING THERE

From I-15, take Exit 6 (Bluff Street/UT 18 North) in St. George. Drive northwest about 11 miles on UT 18 to the park entrance, on your left. The campground is about 2.2 miles south of the park entrance on Snow Canyon Drive, on your left.

GPS COORDINATES: N37° 12.183' W113° 38.447'

49

⛺ Starr Springs Campground

Beauty: ★★★ / Privacy: ★★★★ / Quiet: ★★★★ / Spaciousness: ★★★ / Security: ★★★★ /
Cleanliness: ★★★★

Sneak down to Glen Canyon NRA during the day for some of its overlooked hikes.

With dollar signs in his eyes, a hopeful Al Starr came to the southern tip of the Henry Mountains in the 1880s in search of mining fortunes. Instead, Starr was met with a cruel reminder of how unforgiving the untamed west can be. His mine never produced any ore, and he was forced to close down the operation when drought and locoweed (a toxic plant that wreaks havoc on an animal's nervous system) killed most of his horses.

Today conditions are much more hospitable at Starr Springs, although there are still reminders, besides the campground's name, of Starr's misfortune. Just before arriving at camp, you'll see the remnants of a small structure on the left-hand side of the road. A sign there recounts this woeful tale of a once-hopeful miner. The structure was to be the base of his operations, though Starr was defeated by the desert before his buildings could be completed.

Starr Springs Campground is arranged in a single loop of 12 individual sites numbered counterclockwise along the road. Sites 1–5 are surrounded by relatively flat land, while sites 6–8 back up into a gentle downhill slope populated with thick brush. Sites 9–12 return to flat space, but 10 and 11 offer less shade than their counterparts. Still, site 10 is handsome and spacious enough to merit consideration. It's got quick access to water and restroom facilities. Site 5 shares these characteristics and is situated on the inside of the loop.

A handy little day-use area, located just below the campground on the drive in, has several picnic tables and massive cottonwood trees for shade. The main campground is shaded by the resident oak trees, which do a good job of blocking out the intense heat in this part of the state.

Plentiful oak trees help dispel the Utah summer heat.

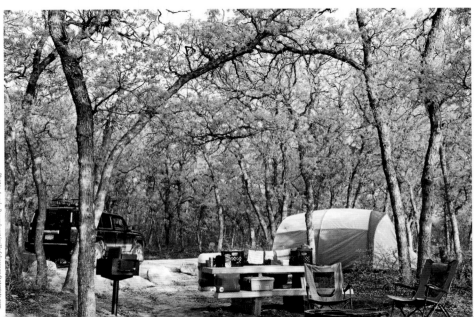

Photo: Angela Rowenhorst/grilledcheeseandtatertots.com

KEY INFORMATION

LOCATION: West of US 276, Lake Powell, UT 84533

CONTACT: 435-542-3461, blm.gov/utah

OPERATED BY: Bureau of Land Management, Henry Mountains Field Station

OPEN: April–November

SITES: 12

EACH SITE: Picnic table, fire ring, barbecue stand

ASSIGNMENT: First-come, first-served; no reservations

REGISTRATION: On-site self-registration

AMENITIES: Vault toilets, water

PARKING: At campsites only

FEE: $4/night

WHEELCHAIR ACCESS: Not designated

ELEVATION: 6,100'

RESTRICTIONS:

PETS: On leash only

FIRES: In fire rings only

ALCOHOL: Permitted

VEHICLES: Large RVs not recommended

OTHER: 14-day stay limit

You'll need to call ahead to the Bureau of Land Management (BLM) to check the status of the drinking water at Starr Springs. The campground is piped for water and has provided service for many years, but there have been problems in the past with the availability of drinking water. The BLM just recently completed some renovations after the campground was damaged by flooding; as of this writing, the water is flowing and there are some new tent pads.

The small Panorama Knoll Nature Trail begins just north of the campground and gives the curious just a taste of what the Henry Mountains offer by showcasing some of the natural wonders and offering a glimpse at the soaring peak of Mount Hillers. To summit the peak, go back down to the main road and continue to wrap around the hillside toward Stanton Pass. From there, it's pretty much a straight shot up the side of the mountain. The hike will compensate you for your efforts with killer views of Capitol Reef National Park's Waterpocket Fold, a 100-mile-long fold in the crust of the earth.

Keep your eyes peeled for the free-roaming bison herd of the Henry Mountains area, but don't be disappointed if they don't make an appearance; instead, focus on the variety of birds in the region, including a slew of different jays, flycatchers, and vireos.

There's no denying that Lake Powell reigns as the region's most popular attraction. The reservoir, encompassed in the larger Glen Canyon Recreation Area, draws around two and a half million visitors each year. There are two ways to do Powell: the loud way or the quiet way. Both have their merits, but if you stay at Starr Springs you're probably more interested in the quiet way. Sneak down to Glen Canyon National Recreation Area during the day for some of its overlooked hikes and side canyon adventures. The park's website (nps.gov/glca) lists many of the day hikes by region, as well as a few of the park's most popular long hikes. Depending on which area you explore, you could be the only human being for miles. After a day of tranquil hiking, pass by the crowds in the closer campgrounds on your way back to the cooler and more comfortable campground you left that morning.

The loud way—by powerboat, houseboat, or in one of the campgrounds right on the camp's shore—is really a riot. Most Powell devotees do it this way and still manage to fit in a bit of quiet time in one of the fingerlike side canyons the reservoir is famous for. If you're the kind of person who wants to be right in the middle of the action, you'll probably be happier at one of the campgrounds closer to the water.

When most people think of the Henry Mountains, Lake Powell, or Glen Canyon, they don't think of Starr Springs Campground. Use that to your advantage for an unorthodox tent trip to southern Utah's summer recreation headquarters.

Starr Springs Campground

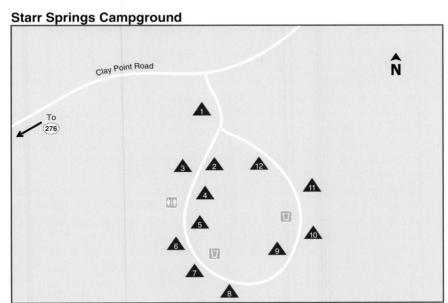

GETTING THERE

From the intersection of UT 24 and UT 95 in Hanksville, drive 26 miles southeast on UT 95. Turn right (south) onto UT 276 and drive 21 miles. Turn right at the brown campground sign, and continue almost 4 miles on a graded dirt road to the campground.

GPS COORDINATES: N37° 50.951' W110° 39.794'

50

Zion National Park:
LAVA POINT CAMPGROUND

Beauty: ★★★★ / Privacy: ★★★ / Quiet: ★★★★★ / Spaciousness: ★★★★ / Security: ★★★★★ /
Cleanliness: ★★★★

Zion means "refuge" or "sanctuary," and that's exactly what Lava Point is.

Perched high in the Kolob Terrace section of Zion National Park is the quiet and unassuming Lava Point Campground. Few people venture to this section of the park, and those who do aren't visiting by accident. Lava Point is where serious park visitors, especially hikers, make camp. It's the capital of the *other* Zion National Park.

While countless campers clog the crowded streets near the Zion Canyon Visitor Center, Lava Point remains blissfully unaware. As you make the turnoff onto Kolob Road Terrace near the town of Virgin, you get the feeling that you know something no one else does. The turn is not well marked, and the road passes through a small residential area before ascending along North Creek.

Climbing along the creek, you'll enter and exit park boundaries two separate times. It's easy to tell when a boundary has been crossed, as the road changes color: Zion roads are red-hued asphalt, and state roads are black. The changing colors beneath you, however, pale in comparison to the changing colors of the environment around you. Your 4,000-foot ascent will take you from scrubby brown-and-olive bushes through thick, light-green trees; around massive, bulbous gray-and-tan rock knobs; and near high-plateau farms. Near the end of the 30-mile road, you'll see a bright-blue reservoir and find Lava Point Campground.

Zion is a Hebrew word meaning "refuge" or "sanctuary," and that's exactly what Zion's Lava Point is. It's a small, single-loop campground with just six primitive sites only open during summer, boasting views that will knock your socks off. This is an aspen-guarded refuge from the 2.5 million visitors who come to Zion each year.

The campsites here are flat and mostly shaded, with convenient garbage service and adequate space to spread out your things. The sites are set a bit too close together, but the

A view of Zion Canyon and the Virgin River from the West Rim Trail

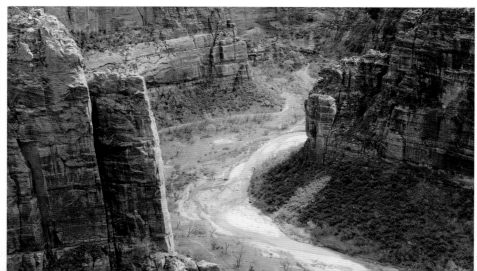

KEY INFORMATION

LOCATION: Lava Point Road off Kolob Terrace Road, Springdale, UT 84767-1099

CONTACT: 435-772-3256, nps.gov/zion

OPERATED BY: Zion National Park, National Park Service

OPEN: June–October (depending on weather)

SITES: 6

EACH SITE: Picnic table, fire ring, garbage can

ASSIGNMENT: First-come, first-served; no reservations

REGISTRATION: On-site self-registration

AMENITIES: Vault toilets, garbage service

PARKING: At campsites only

FEE: None to camp; $30 park entrance fee required. See nps.gov/zion/planyourvisit/fees.htm for more information.

WHEELCHAIR ACCESS: Not designated

ELEVATION: 7,870'

RESTRICTIONS:

PETS: On leash only

FIRES: In fire rings only

ALCOHOL: Permitted

VEHICLES: Up to 19 feet

OTHER: 14-day stay limit in season, additional 30 days/year off-season; maximum 6 people, 2 vehicles, 3 tents/site

---

quiet in the surrounding air is contagious, and most campers can't help but speak in reverent whispers. The loudest noise you're bound to hear on your visit may be the buzzing of flies and other pesky bugs—bring plenty of spray or even a head net. At Lava Point, these insects thrive for most of the summer and can quickly drive you mad.

Next to the camp is the Lava Point Overlook, from which you'll get gorgeous views of the Horse Pasture Plateau as it fades from pine and white fir to juniper and short shrubs. The views have been enhanced by an aggressive restoration project undertaken to reduce the number of invasive white fir trees and help reestablish the aspen population.

Most visitors to Lava Point come with one hike in mind: the West Rim Trail. This 14-mile (one-way) trail connects Lava Point and the Kolob Terrace section of the park with the main canyon, passing views of many side canyons like Potato Hollow and the Great West Canyon, and passing through Refrigerator Canyon. This hike is usually done over two days. Trying to complete it in one just means you won't have time to take all the photos you'd like—a serious mistake on this trail.

Make sure that you acquire the proper permits before heading out on any hike. Because of the park's popularity, permits are required for all overnight trips, all thru-hikes of the Narrows and its tributaries, and several other widely used hikes in the park. Permits for the most popular hikes—The Subway and Mystery Canyon—are distributed only by lottery. For more information, see zionpermits.nps.gov; read this website thoroughly when planning a visit, and always have a backup plan in case you can't get a permit for the area you'd like to hike in.

Recreation isn't bound to park-related attractions. Just 3 miles from Lava Point is Kolob Reservoir, a special-regulations fishery that produces some impressive cutthroat trout. Early-morning and pre-dusk fishing seem to be the key here, although with the right fly you could catch your limit at practically any hour. Just be sure to take paved Kolob Terrace Road all the way to the end to find Kolob Reservoir. Blue Springs Reservoir, just after the turnoff for the campground, may look alluring, but private-cabin owners are quite adamant about keeping it private.

If you're staying at Lava Point for several days, just give in and visit the main canyon area along UT 9. Be aware that in summer the area is accessible by shuttle bus only and can take some time to explore. Crowds aside, hiking through the Virgin River in the main canyon is a fun way to spend an afternoon. Depths range from "sloshy shoes" to "over your head." You'll definitely have to be on your toes.

For a real gut-check, try the Angel's Landing Trail. Acrophobes need not attempt this skinny trail with chain handrails. It takes hikers 1,700 feet up a rugged red knob and leaves them with dizzying, adrenaline-enhanced views.

Zion National Park is the busiest of all Utah national parks, but you'd never know it from staying at Lava Point. Here, the cacophony of cars and tourists is replaced by the quaking of aspen leaves and the quiet of the *other* Zion National Park.

Zion National Park: Lava Point Campground

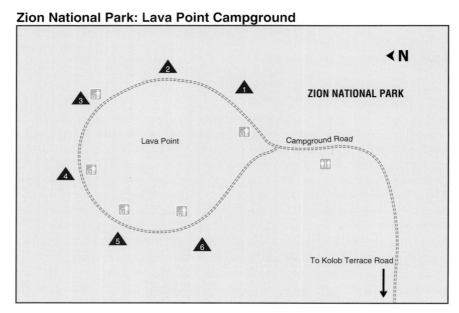

GETTING THERE

Zion National Park is about 300 miles south of Salt Lake City. From I-15, take Exit 27 and head south on UT 17. In 5.9 miles, turn left (east) onto UT 9 in the town of La Verkin. In 6.2 miles, turn left onto Kolob Terrace Road in the town of Virgin and, in 0.8 mile, bear left at the T to continue north on this road. In 6.8 miles, bear right at another intersection to continue north on Kolob Terrace Road; in 4.5 miles, bear right at a third intersection to continue north on this road. In 8 miles, just before Blue Springs Reservoir, turn right at the brown sign for Zion National Park onto Lava Point Road, a dirt road heading southeast. (*Note:* Vehicles longer than 19 feet are prohibited on this road.) In 0.9 mile, keep right (straight) at the intersection to continue on Lava Point Road. In another 0.5 mile, look for the campground entrance on your left.

GPS COORDINATES: N37° 23.000' W113° 1.976'

APPENDIX A:

CAMPING-EQUIPMENT CHECKLIST

Camping is more fun when you can enjoy it at a moment's notice. You never know when the opportunity may arise to head for the hills, and when it does, wouldn't it be nice to be able to pack your car with all the essentials drawn from prepacked boxes carefully cleaned, resupplied, and stored after your last trip?

COOKING/KITCHEN

(Packed in a plastic box)
Bowls
Can opener
Cooking pots with lids
Cooler
Dishcloth and towel
Dishpan
Dry-food box
Dutch oven and fire pan
5-gallon water jug
Flatwear
Frying pan
Insulated plastic mugs
Large serving spoon
Lighter or matches
Paper towels
Plates
Pocketknife
Rain tarp or dining fly
Sharp knife
Spatula
Spices, salt, pepper
Stove and fuel
Strainer
Tablecloth
Tinfoil
Trash bags
Wooden spoon

SLEEPING QUARTERS

Ground cloth
Pillow
Sleeping bag
Sleeping pad
Tent and rainfly

MISCELLANEOUS

Candles
Day pack
Extra batteries
Firewood
First aid kit
Flashlight
Folding camp chair
Lantern
Maps
Premoistened towelettes
Resealable plastic bags
Saw/ax
Toilet paper
Water bottles

EXTRAS

Binoculars
Books
Camera
Cards and games
Field guides
Fishing rod
Frisbee

APPENDIX B:

SOURCES OF INFORMATION

NATIONAL PARK SERVICE
nps.gov

ARCHES NATIONAL PARK
PO Box 907
Moab, UT 84532
435-719-2299
nps.gov/arch

BRYCE CANYON NATIONAL PARK
PO Box 640201
Bryce Canyon, UT 84764-0201
435-834-5322
nps.gov/brca

CANYONLANDS NATIONAL PARK
2282 SW Resource Blvd.
Moab, UT 84532
435-719-2313
nps.gov/cany

CAPITOL REEF NATIONAL PARK
HC 70, Box 15
Torrey, UT 84775
435-425-3791, Ext. 111
nps.gov/care

NATURAL BRIDGES NATIONAL MONUMENT
HC 60, Box 1
Lake Powell, UT 84533
435-692-1234
nps.gov/nabr

ZION NATIONAL PARK
1 Zion Park Blvd. (UT 9)
Springdale, UT 84767
435-772-3256
nps.gov/zion

U.S. FOREST SERVICE
www.fs.usda.gov

ASHLEY NATIONAL FOREST
355 N. Vernal Ave.
Vernal, UT 84078
435-789-1181
www.fs.usda.gov/ashley

DIXIE NATIONAL FOREST
1789 N. Wedgewood Lane
Cedar City, UT 84720
435-865-3700
www.fs.usda.gov/dixie

FISHLAKE NATIONAL FOREST
115 E. 900 N.
Richfield, UT 84701
435-896-9233
www.fs.usda.gov/fishlake

MANTI–LA SAL NATIONAL FOREST
599 W. Price River Drive
Price, UT 84501
435-637-2817
www.fs.usda.gov/mantilasal

SAWTOOTH NATIONAL FOREST
2647 Kimberly Road E.
Twin Falls, ID 83301
208-737-3200
www.fs.usda.gov/sawtooth

UINTA-WASATCH-CACHE NATIONAL FOREST
125 S. State St.
Salt Lake City, UT 84138
801-236-3400
www.fs.usda.gov/uwcnf

OTHER RESOURCES

BUREAU OF LAND MANAGEMENT, UTAH STATE OFFICE
blm.gov/utah

Henry Mountains Field Office
380 S. 100 W.
Hanksville, UT 84734
435-542-3461

Moab Field Office
82 E. Dogwood St.
Moab, UT 84532
435-259-2106

Monticello Field Office
365 N. Main St.
Monticello, UT 84535
435-587-1500

St. George Field Office
345 E. Riverside Drive
St. George, UT 84101
435-688-3200

Salt Lake Field Office
2370 S. Decker Lake Blvd.
West Valley, UT 84101
801-977-4397

CALTOPO
(Online topographic maps)
caltopo.com

PUBLIC LANDS INTERPRETIVE ASSOCIATION
(Online directory of U.S. Forest Service, Bureau of Land Management, and U.S. Fish and Wildlife Service lands in the western United States, plus maps, books, gifts, and more)
publiclands.org

U.S. GEOLOGICAL SURVEY
(Maps, recreational passes, and more)
store.usgs.gov

UTAH STATE PARKS
1594 W. North Temple
Salt Lake City, UT 84116
801-538-7220
stateparks.utah.gov

UTAH DIVISION OF WILDLIFE RESOURCES
1594 W. North Temple
Salt Lake City, UT 84116
801-538-4700
wildlife.utah.gov

INDEX

campground locator map, iv; about, 3

campground profiles, 3

campgrounds. *See also specific campground*
    best, by category, x–xi
    GPS entrance coordinates, 3
    individual ratings, 1–3
    in Northern Utah, 12–90
    reserving sites, 7
    in Southern Utah, 105–164
    in Western Utah, 92–103

camping-equipment checklist, 165

Canyonlands National Park, 127
    contact information, 166
    Hamburger Rock Campground, 114–16

Capitol Reef fruit, 117–18

Capitol Reef National Park, 113, 130, 150
    contact information, 166
    Fruita Campground, 117–19

Capitol Reef National Park's Waterpocket Fold, 160

Caribou-Targhee National Forest, 92, 94

Carmel Canyon Trail, 134

Carter Creek, 34

Cassidy, Butch, 42

Castle Valley, 147–48

Cathedral Valley, 118, 130

catholes, 8

Causey Reservoir, 25

Cedar Breaks National Monument, 113, 120, 121

Cedar Canyon Campground, 120–22

Cedar City, 120

cell phones, 9

Cecret Lake Trail, 12

checklist, camping-equipment, 165

Clark Lake, 148

Cleanliness (ratings), 2–3

cleanliness, best campgrounds for, xi

Clear Creek Campground, 92–94

clothing, 7

Clover Spring Campground, 95–97

Coffee Peak, 62

Colorado Plateau, 118, 154

Colorado River, 105, 107, 124, 140, 147

cougars (mountain lions), 5, 96

Cowboy Camp Campground, 123–25

Crow Creek, 120, 121

Crystal Lake, 31

Curtis Bench Trail, 134

D

Dalton Springs Campground, 126–28

Dead Horse Point State Park, 124

Deep Creek Campground, 33–35

Deep Creek Canyon, 46

Deep Creek Lake, 130

Deep Creek Mountains, 103

Deer Creek Lake, 152

Delicate Arch, 106

Deseret Peak, 97, 99

Deseret Peak Wilderness, 98–99

Devil's Kitchen, 73

Diamond Fork Canyon, 36–37

Dick's, 32

Dixie National Forest, 122, 145, 150

Donut Falls, 77

Dowd Mountain Overlook and Picnic Area, 43

drinking water, 9

Dry Canyon Campground, 36–38

Dry Creek Canyon Trail, 22

Dry Fork–Beaver Basin Trail, 149

Duchesne River, 65

E

Electric Lake, 41

elk, 47, 53, 70–71, 84

Elkhorn Campground, 129–131

Elkhorn Lake, 130

Entrada Canyon Trail, 134

equipment, camping checklist, 165

Escalante Petrified Forest State Park, 113

F

family-friendly campgrounds, xi

Farmington Canyon, 27

Fielding Garr Ranch, 17

Fiery Furnace, 106

Fifth Water Hot Springs, 37

fires, 9

snakes, 6
Snow Canyon State Park Campground, 156–58
Soldier Creek Dam, 19
Solitude Mountain Resort, 13, 77
South Willow Canyon, 99, 100
South Willow Lake, 99
Southern Utah campgrounds, 105–164
spaciousness, best campgrounds for, x
Spanish Fork Canyon, 36
Spirit Creek, 146
Spirit Lake, 34
Squaw Peak, 48
Stansbury Mountains, 98, 99, 100
star rating system, 1–3
Starr, Al, 159
Starr Springs Campground, 159–161
Steadman, Jeffrey, viii, 179
Steep Creek Lake, 152
Strawberry Marina, 20
Strawberry Point Trailhead, 122
Strawberry Reservoir, 18, 19
streams, crossing, 10
Stuart Visitor Information Center, 40
Subway, The, 163
Survey Lake, ix, 90

T

Tanners Flat Campground, 79–81
Temple Quarry Nature Trail, 81
tents, pitching, 7
Thousand Lake Mountain, 119, 129, 130, 131
Tibble Fork Reservoir, 82, 84
ticks, 6
Timpanogos Cave National Monument, 84
Timpooneke Campground, 82–84
toilets, 7–8
Tony Grove Campground, 85–87
Tony Grove Lake, 46, 85, 86, 87
trash, 9
Twin Lakes, 77

U

Uinta Mountains, 30–31, 32, 33, 51
Uinta-Wasatch-Cache National Forest, 28, 54, 64, 73, 74, 78, 85, 88, 92

Upper Red Pine Lake, 81
Upper Stillwater Reservoir, 88
Utah Fishing Guidebook, 52, 70
Utah State Parks, 167

V

Vernon Reservoir, 97
Virgin River Rim Trail, 122

W

Waddell, William B., 101
Wardsworth Creek, 22
Warner Lake, 149
Wasatch Front, 19, 65, 95
Wasatch Mountain Lodge, 77
Wasatch Mountain Range, 80, 99
Wasatch Wildflower Festival, 13
water, drinking, 9
Waterpocket Fold, Capitol Reef National Park, 160
weather, 3–4
Weir Lake, 31
West Desert, 96, 101, 102, 103
West Rim Trail, 162, 163
Western Utah campgrounds, 92–103
wheelchairs, best campgrounds for, xi
whistles, 10
White Canyon, 46
White Pine Lake, 81, 86
Willow Lakes Trail, 99
Witt, Greg, 84
Wolfe Ranch, 106
Woodruff Creek Reservoir, 67
Woods Ranch Recreation Area, 122

Y

Yellowpine Campground, 88–90
Young, Brigham, 15

Z

Zion National Park, 145
    contact information, 166
    Lava Point Campground, 162–64

ABOUT THE AUTHOR

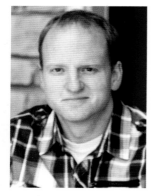

Jeffrey Steadman was born and raised in Utah, which he began appreciating shortly after leaving the womb. As a child, he spent his summers exploring the canyons of the Wasatch Front on family hikes. These days, he explores all that Utah has to offer in every season.

He has slept in snow caves, has been caught in lightning storms at 12,000 feet, and has occasionally been known to catch fish from streams with his bare hands.

Jeffrey is an accomplished writer who enjoys introducing new campers to the outdoors through youth volunteer programs, classroom instruction, and planning giant camping trips with new friends.

When he's not in the backcountry, he enjoys cooking, gardening, photography, and spending time with family. He lives near Salt Lake City with Mountain Jane, a wirehaired pointing griffon who just can't get enough camping.

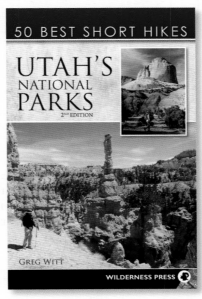
 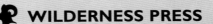 WILDERNESS PRESS

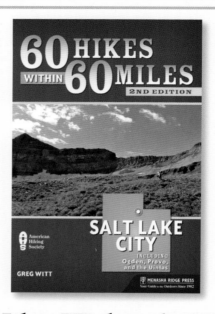
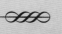 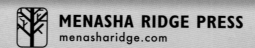

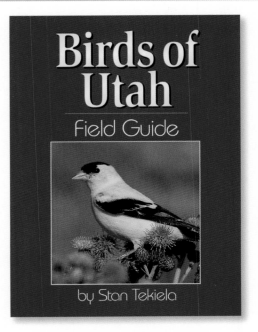

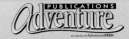

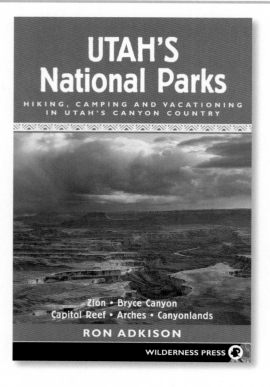
  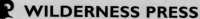

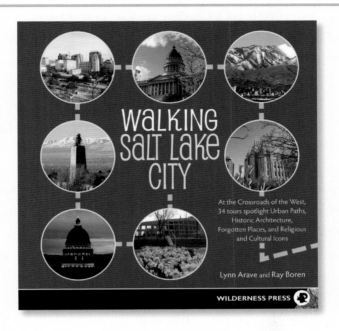

DEAR CUSTOMERS AND FRIENDS,

SUPPORTING YOUR INTEREST IN OUTDOOR ADVENTURE, travel, and an active lifestyle is central to our operations, from the authors we choose to the locations we detail to the way we design our books. Menasha Ridge Press was incorporated in 1982 by a group of veteran outdoorsmen and professional outfitters. For many years now, we've specialized in creating books that benefit the outdoors enthusiast.

Almost immediately, Menasha Ridge Press earned a reputation for revolutionizing outdoors- and travel-guidebook publishing. For such activities as canoeing, kayaking, hiking, backpacking, and mountain biking, we established new standards of quality that transformed the whole genre, resulting in outdoor-recreation guides of great sophistication and solid content. Menasha Ridge Press continues to be outdoor publishing's greatest innovator.

The folks at Menasha Ridge Press are as at home on a whitewater river or mountain trail as they are editing a manuscript. The books we build for you are the best they can be, because we're responding to your needs. Plus, we use and depend on them ourselves.

We look forward to seeing you on the river or the trail. If you'd like to contact us directly, visit us at menasharidge.com. We thank you for your interest in our books and the natural world around us all.

SAFE TRAVELS,

Bob Sehlinger

BOB SEHLINGER
PUBLISHER